100 Questions & Answers About Chronic Illness

Robert A. Norman, DO, MPH, MBA

Chief Physician and Owner, Dermatology Health Care
Tampa, FL
Associate Clinical Professor, Dermatology
Nova Southeastern University
College of Medical Sciences
Fort Lauderdale, FL

Linda Ruescher

Editor and Facilitator Coordinator
Lupus Foundation of America
Greater Florida Chapter
St. Petersburg, FL
Master Trainer
Chronic Disease Self-Management Program
Patient Education in the Department of Medicine
Stanford University
Palo Alto, CA

JONES AND BARTLETT PUBLISHERS
Sudbury, Massachusetts
BOSTON   TORONTO   LONDON   SINGAPORE

5318010

World Headquarters
Jones and Bartlett Publishers
40 Tall Pine Drive
Sudbury, MA 01776
978-443-5000
info@jbpub.com
www.jbpub.com

Jones and Bartlett Publishers
Canada
6339 Ormindale Way
Mississauga, Ontario L5V 1J2
Canada

Jones and Bartlett Publishers
International
Barb House, Barb Mews
London W6 7PA
United Kingdom

Jones and Bartlett's books and products are available through most bookstores and online book-sellers. To contact Jones and Bartlett Publishers directly, call 800-832-0034, fax 978-443-8000, or visit our website, www.jbpub.com.

Substantial discounts on bulk quantities of Jones and Bartlett's publications are available to corporations, professional associations, and other qualified organizations. For details and specific discount information, contact the special sales department at Jones and Bartlett via the above contact information or send an email to specialsales@jbpub.com.

The authors, editor, and publisher have made every effort to provide accurate information. However, they are not responsible for errors, omissions, or for any outcomes related to the use of the contents of this book and take no responsibility for the use of the products and procedures described. Treatments and side effects described in this book may not be applicable to all people; likewise, some people may require a dose or experience a side effect that is not described herein. Drugs and medical devices are discussed that may have limited availability controlled by the Food and Drug Administration (FDA) for use only in a research study or clinical trial. Research, clinical practice, and government regulations often change the accepted standard in this field. When consideration is being given to use of any drug in the clinical setting, the health care provider or reader is responsible for determining FDA status of the drug, reading the package insert, and reviewing prescribing information for the most up-to-date recommendations on dose, precautions, and contraindications, and determining the appropriate usage for the product. This is especially important in the case of drugs that are new or seldom used.

Production Credits
Executive Publisher: Christopher Davis
Editorial Assistant: Sara Cameron
Associate Production Editor: Sarah Bayle
Senior Marketing Manager: Barb Bartoszek
Manufacturing and Inventory Control Supervisor:
 Amy Bacus

Composition: Glyph International
Cover Design: Carolyn Downer
Cover Image: © DNF-Style Photography/
 ShutterStock, Inc.
Printing and Binding: Malloy, Inc.
Cover Printing: Malloy, Inc.

Library of Congress Cataloging-in-Publication Data
Norman, Robert A., 1955-
 100 questions & answers about chronic illness / Robert A. Norman, Linda
Ruescher.
  p. cm.
 Includes index.
 ISBN 978-0-7637-7764-7 (alk. paper)
 1. Chronic diseases—Popular works. 2. Chronic diseases—Miscellanea. I. Ruescher,
Linda. II. Title. III. Title: One hundred questions & answers about chronic illness. IV. Title:
100 questions and answers about chronic illness.
 RC108.N67 2010
 616'.044—dc22

2009039587

6048

Printed in the United States of America
13 12 11 10 09   10 9 8 7 6 5 4 3 2 1

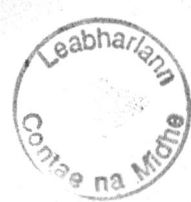

More Praise for *100 Questions & Answers About Chronic Illness*

"In 20 years of working with patients coping with chronic illness, this is the best all-encompassing guide I have come across to assist those navigating the challenges of the symptoms, treatments, and medical maze of decisions that come with the package when one is diagnosed with a chronic illness such as lupus, multiple sclerosis, arthritis, or other autoimmune diseases. Written with great knowledge and compassion, and based on her own personal journey and those of the many people she has helped along that path, Linda Ruescher and Dr. Rob Norman empower us with in-depth information that can banish the fear and confusion of chronic illness. This book is a must-have for anyone coping with chronic illness. It is a whole toolkit of coping skills, strategies, and valuable information that I am anxious to share with my patients and friends. Dr. Rob Norman and Linda Ruescher put the heart and soul in this difficult and sometimes painful journey from 'patient' to 'person'!"

Patricia Burkett, PsyD, is a clinical psychologist with 20 years of experience specializing in medical psychology practice with pain management, chronic illness, and cancer patients and their families. She is currently associated with Gulfcoast Oncology Associates in St. Petersburg, Florida.

Contents

Part 1: The Basics   1

Questions 1–6 answer basic questions about chronic illness:

- What is chronic illness?
- What causes chronic illness?
- How is the treatment of chronic illness different from the treatment of acute illness?

Part 2: Stages of Grieving   11

Questions 7–18 deal with some of the difficult emotions that arise after a diagnosis of chronic illness:

- Did I cause my disease?
- If I'm never going to get better, why bother trying?
- How can I manage depression?

Part 3: How Chronic Illness Affects Social Relationships   25

Questions 19–24 address the impact of chronic illness on relationships with loved ones, family, and friends:

- Why do I feel so isolated?
- How can I make other people understand what I am going through?
- Should I tell people about my condition?

Part 4: Chronic Illness and the Law   37

Questions 25–30 explain the rights and protections that the law provides for chronically ill and disabled people:

- What rights do I have under the Americans with Disabilities Act?
- What is the Family Medical Leave Act, and how does it affect me?
- How can I be sure that my wishes will be honored if I am unable to make medical decisions for myself?

Contents

The demand for answers about chronic care is increasing rapidly, especially as the population ages. Many people throughout the world are living well into their old age. By the time many of us reach middle age, we have at least one, if not three or four, chronic problems. The collection often includes obesity, hypertension, and back pain. For those who have been unfortunate in the genetic lottery, other problems such as diabetes (which affects 8% of the U.S. population), lupus, or psoriasis may add to the illness burden.

In the United States alone, more than 133 million suffer from asthma, depression, and other chronic conditions. The infectious diseases that plagued many people during the last century have taken a back seat to the long-term management of many illnesses. Many of the diseases that began as acute illnesses have now evolved into diseases of chronic care—most notably AIDS. Although we provide a huge amount of acute treatments in our society, the trend is toward chronic care and quality-of-life issues. This book provides support and guidelines, expertise, and references.

The demand is clear—we need to shift from a reactive healthcare system into one that keeps us healthy for as long as possible, and the answers provided here will help you to achieve these goals.

The human body is quite amazing, but it is prone to breakdown. The study of chronic illness can help us appreciate our marvelous body and mind when they are working at their best. We have to optimize what we have been given, and this book is designed to help you achieve your best life—*100 Questions & Answers About Chronic Illness* outlines chronic care and what you can do to improve what you have. We hope that your pain and problems, as well as your healthcare costs, can lessen if you use the advice in this book.

The modern media has changed and often warped our perceptions of ourselves. It seems as if every new magazine and TV commercial is filled with drugs and devices that promise a renewed life and pain-free living. We need more accurate advice to cut through the enormous load of information on chronic care that comes at us from every direction. This book provides the latest in treatments and gives you the most important tools to help deal with various chronic maladies.

We have seen and dealt with many of these illnesses and certainly have heard many of the associated problems and concerns—Dr. Norman in his role as physician, and Ms. Ruescher as director of support groups for the Lupus Foundation and as a lupus patient herself. We both believe there is a paucity of information on chronic care and have been passionate about writing this book and giving you a springboard to search for more answers to your questions. A delay in recognition and treatment can lead to a decreased quality of life and more misery. Often there are not enough informed providers and specialists with the time to provide the information and resources we include here.

Our goal is to offer a guide to understanding what happens in chronic care conditions and to emphasize that you have enormous opportunities to improve your general health by following the suggestions we have included. For more help with your own comprehensive prevention and treatment, it is important to consult with your local physician and to check the reputable online sites, some of which have been included here.

Peace,

Dr. Robert Norman and Linda Ruescher

Dr. Krokowski, "Do you come as a patient, may I ask?"

Hans Castorp replied, mentioning his examination and his 3-week visit, and ended by saying he was, thank God, perfectly healthy.

"Really?" asked Krokowski, putting his head teasingly on one side. His smile grew broader. "Then you are a phenomenon worthy of study. I, for one, have never in my life come across a perfectly healthy human being."

Thomas Mann, *The Magic Mountain*

We live in a time when health care is complicated and frustrating. In the world of medical practice, we have shifted from a simple, personal interaction with the patient to a "hurry up" managed care, bureaucratic, defensive, complicated mess. Naturally, it is shocking and overwhelming to accept and understand the diagnosis of a chronic illness. What should I expect? Why me? How is my life going to change? Suddenly, many diverse questions come to mind and very few answers. This journey of uncertainties becomes less stressful when traveled with empathetic caring from charismatic healthcare providers.

As a physician in private practice for over 13 years, caring for patients with chronic illnesses, I am well aware that miracle cures are few and far between. Long ago, I settled into the role of provider not only of patient care, but also information regarding alternative treatment options and, most importantly, hope.

I have known Linda Ruescher for over 8 years, initially as her physician who diagnosed her with a terrible chronic illness called systemic lupus. She has demonstrated to me that health is much more than the absence of illness. As a lupus patient and the director of support groups for the Lupus Foundation of America, Greater Florida Chapter, Ms. Ruescher has been passionate about the promotion of body/mind to heal and improve itself. This book is a self-help manual of frequently asked questions and answers, as well as a practical recommendation with real resources available in any community for patients newly diagnosed with a chronic illness. My heartfelt gratitude goes out to Ms. Ruescher and Dr. Robert Norman for their great effort to provide encouragement and for the diligent effort taken to produce this book. Great job!

Sincerely and respectfully,
Edgard Janer, MD

Acknowledgments

Our heartfelt thanks to Nancy Duffy for her gentle guidance in bringing this book to fruition. We also thank the staff at Jones and Bartlett, especially Sarah Bayle and Sara Cameron, for their hard work on this project. We are indebted to the many patients whose struggles and concerns about living with chronic illness taught us so much.

Linda extends special thanks to the members of her medical team—Dr. Edgard Janer, Dr. Alexander Sonkin, and Dr. Ramesh Shah—for their compassionate care, for being true partners in managing lupus, and for their support and encouragement.

PART ONE

The Basics

What is chronic illness?

What causes chronic illness?

How is the treatment of chronic illness
different from the treatment of acute illness?

More . . .

1. What is chronic illness?

A chronic illness is an illness that lasts for a very long time, sometimes for a person's entire life. Chronic illnesses usually develop slowly, often over the course of several years. Symptoms may come and go, varying in intensity, making many chronic illnesses difficult to diagnose. In fact, some patients search for years for an accurate diagnosis. Chronic illnesses may be progressive, getting worse over time when left untreated, like **coronary artery disease** or type 2 **diabetes**. Other diseases like lupus and **Crohn's disease** have periods of activity and periods of relative calm. The majority of chronic illnesses have no cure. Even though there is no cure, chronic illnesses still need to be treated. The goals of treatment are to manage symptoms, prevent permanent damage, and stop or slow the progression of the disease. Some diseases like **HIV/AIDS** and cancer are gradually shifting away from being a death sentence to becoming chronic conditions.

Acute illnesses, on the other hand, have a clear beginning, climax, and resolution. Think about the common cold. You begin to feel sick. Your nose gets stuffy. You feel tired and achy. You cough, and your throat hurts. You run a fever. When the cold is at its worst, you go to bed. You sleep a lot, the fever breaks, and you begin to feel better. Soon you are back to normal with no lasting problems. Some acute illnesses pass with time while others can be cured with medication. In cases of acute illness, patients recover and return to normal (most of them) or they die.

2. Who gets chronic illness?

According to the Robert Wood Johnson Foundation, more than 133 million Americans have chronic medical conditions—that's more than 16 times the entire

---

A chronic illness is an illness that lasts for a very long time, sometimes for a person's entire life.

Coronary artery disease

Disease of the blood vessels that involves the heart.

Diabetes (types 1 and 2)

Diabetes occurs when the body is not able to keep blood sugar balanced. Type 1 diabetes is autoimmune. Type 2 diabetes develops as a result of obesity, lifestyle, or age.

Crohn's disease

A chronic inflammatory disease affecting the digestive tract.

HIV/AIDS

A virus-induced disorder of the immune system whereby a person loses the ability to fight infection.

population of New York City! Why is the number so high? There is no single answer to that question. The answer lies in a number of developments in our world and in medicine.

A century ago, people developed many of the chronic illnesses we see today. But a century ago, many of these diseases had not yet been identified. People got sick and died from many of the same things they get sick from today, but they were not diagnosed and not treated. People simply died or lived miserable lives. Today, with the explosion of knowledge in science and medicine, chronic illnesses are diagnosed, and therefore treated, earlier. Whether or not we have a higher percentage of our population suffering from chronic conditions today than we did in past years is impossible to say. What we do know is that we seem to have more people who are ill because we are now able to diagnose them.

Along with an increase in the ability to make accurate and earlier diagnoses, researchers have also brought us better ways to control these conditions. Because better treatments are available, more people with chronic illness are living longer. As more people live longer, there will be a higher identified segment of the population living with chronic illness and disability. For example, a person diagnosed with systemic lupus 25 years ago would have a life expectancy of less than 5 years after diagnosis. Now, the majority of lupus patients who follow their treatment plan can expect to live a relatively normal life span.

Other, more obvious factors contribute to the large numbers of people with chronic illness. **Obesity** has become an epidemic in the United States, leading to cardiovascular disease and diabetes. The stress of "civilized" society is a direct factor in the development

Obesity

Overweight and obesity are both labels for ranges of weight that are greater than what is generally considered healthy for a given height. An adult who has a body mass index (BMI) between 25 and 29.9 is considered overweight. An adult who has a BMI of 30 or higher is considered obese.

of countless diseases. Add to obesity and stress things like inadequate nutrition, lack of exercise, environmental pollutants, chemicals in food and water, smoking, and alcohol or drugs and it's easy to see why the number of chronically ill people is so high. And don't forget that the population is generally getting older as baby boomers age. With a larger percentage of the population becoming elderly, the percentage of people with chronic illness in the general population will go up. But chronic illness can strike at any age.

3. What causes chronic illness?

The causes of some chronic illnesses have been identified. According to the American Academy of Family Physicians, "Most chronic illnesses develop long before the physician learns about their symptoms. Over time, genetics, lifestyle choices, psychological pressure, exposure to chemicals, other environmental hazards, and inappropriate medications, as well as other factors, contribute to the eventual manifestation of the condition." Although genetics are beyond our control, many of the other risk factors are within our control.

The causes of other chronic illnesses are still a mystery. Autoimmune diseases are increasing at an alarming rate. According to the American Autoimmune Related Diseases Association, 23.5 million Americans have autoimmune conditions, making these diseases the leading cause of chronic illness. There are over 100 autoimmune diseases! No one has been able to pinpoint what makes a person's immune system go haywire and attack the healthy self.

As scientists uncover risk factors for chronic illnesses, we can become more and more proactive in preventing them. As more causes for chronic illnesses are discovered, treatments will improve and cures may be discovered. Just as HIV/AIDS has moved from terminal to chronic for most patients, so will some chronic conditions move to curable.

Linda R's comment:

I got sick every year around Christmas time. I would hope whatever it was that made me so tired and achy would go away with time. Most years there was no improvement until after Easter. At first I went to doctors, but the answer was always the same. They told me I had a virus or something that was going around. There was really nothing they could do. I was working too hard and should take a week or so off. They prescribed high doses of ibuprofen and sent me on my way. After a while, I stopped looking for answers and just toughed it out. Maybe I was just a weak person. Maybe it was all in my head. Finally, I got so sick that a friend had to call an ambulance. It took just over 1 week in the hospital before I finally got a diagnosis!

4. Why are so many chronic illnesses difficult to diagnose?

Chronic illnesses develop slowly over a period of time. Symptoms come and go, leaving patients wondering if something is really wrong or if it's all in their head. When these patients finally do report symptoms to their doctors, the disease has usually been present for some time. By the time a patient gets in to see the doctor, the symptoms may have subsided, leaving the doctor wondering if it's all in the patient's head. It's like the car owner who notices a strange noise in the car, only to have it disappear when the car is taken to the mechanic, or like the toothache that disappears when you walk into the dentist's office. Medications may have been prescribed that masked the symptoms without ever getting to the root cause of the disease.

People who have one chronic condition usually have others, making diagnosis even more difficult.

Hypertension
High blood pressure.

By the time both the patient and the doctor are convinced that something is wrong, permanent damage may have already occurred. People who have one chronic condition usually have others, making diagnosis even more difficult. For example, a patient with a bad lipid profile probably also suffers from obesity, diabetes, and **hypertension**. Coming to a diagnosis is even more difficult in diseases where there are no definitive lab tests to identify the disease. In these cases, doctors may arrive at a diagnosis by process of elimination.

Most doctors are trained in acute care. They see the problem, name it, fix it, and send you on your way. According to David Jones, MD, of the Institute for Functional Medicine, medical students are taught to quickly diagnose an illness and provide acute care for the symptoms; medical schools train future physicians for what will be about 20% of their practices, but 78% of today's patients present with at least one chronic illness.

5. How is the treatment of chronic illness different from the treatment of acute illness?

There are three major ways in which the treatment of chronic illness and the treatment of acute illness differ. The first is the goal of treatment. The second is the difference in the relationship between medical professional and patient. The third is the ongoing responsibility of the patient for his or her own health.

If you break your arm (acute condition), the treatment goal is obvious—set the bone, and immobilize the fracture with a cast until healing takes place. The treatment goal is to fix the fracture. If you have an infection caused by bacteria, such as strep throat, the treatment goal is also clear—kill the bacteria. Antibiotics are prescribed and administered. The infection clears, and the patient resumes normal activities.

Since chronic illnesses can't be cured, at least at this point in time, the treatment goals are very different. The goals of treatment in chronic illness are to minimize symptoms, long-term damage, and disease activity. While the course of action to achieve the treatment goals in acute illness is usually pretty clear, that's not usually the case with chronic conditions. People with one chronic disease often have other conditions, making the development of a treatment plan less cut and dried. The **remitting/flaring** nature of many chronic diseases, coupled with the fact that symptoms may change radically over time, make finding the proper course of treatment even more difficult.

Remitting/flaring
Periods of relative calm and periods of increased disease activity.

The second major difference in the treatment of chronic illness versus the treatment of acute illness is the relationship between the medical professional and the patient. In the acute case of a broken bone or an infection, the doctor is the authority, and the treatment is clear. If you are sitting in the emergency room with a bone that is broken or a raging infection, you are not going to negotiate treatment options! You rely on the doctor's expertise and follow the treatment plan without question. In cases of chronic illness, the patient and the medical professional(s) have to work as partners in managing the disease. The patient must learn self-management and become educated about the disease. And since there are no absolutes in the treatment of chronic illness, the patient and professional must develop a good working relationship with open channels of communication. Often, more than one treatment option is available. While you are not likely to debate the need for a cast, if you have a chronic condition you may find yourself debating treatment options with your doctor.

The third difference is in the role of the patient. It is the patient's job to follow the treatment plan faithfully. Medications must be taken as often as prescribed and according to directions. All the medicine in the world won't do any good if it is not taken properly. The patient must monitor symptoms on a daily basis and then be very accurate in reporting those symptoms to the doctor at the next visit. The patient is also responsible for lifestyle changes—rest, exercise, nutrition, and stress management—that can minimize the effects of the disease.

6. How does the doctor-patient relationship in chronic illness differ from the doctor-patient relationship in cases of acute illness?

The doctor-patient relationship in chronic illness is critical in managing the disease. Going back to the example of a broken leg, it doesn't much matter whether you have a relationship with that doctor; you just want the leg set. People with chronic illness see their doctors often, sometimes monthly, and so establishing a good working relationship is essential. Good relationships are based on openness, trust, and good communication.

Doctor and patient must both be open with one another. The relationship will not work if the patient is hiding vital information. That information might be alternative therapies the patient is trying, being honest about not taking medications or following the treatment regimen, disclosing all vitamins and supplements, or engaging in high-risk behaviors. The relationship will not work if the doctor is hiding information about the seriousness of the disease and what the patient can likely expect in the future. Be honest and open with your doctor. Part of being honest and open is making sure that your doctor understands that you expect the same honesty and openness in return.

Trust is essential in any relationship but especially as it applies to doctor and patient. The patient trusts the doctor to have his or her best interest at heart. The patient also trusts the doctor's training and expertise. With the amount of information and misinformation available on the Internet, patients often try to second-guess doctors. Open discussion is good. Believing that the doctor is engaged in a conspiracy to keep you from miracle cures is not. The doctor trusts the patient to report symptoms and changes accurately. The doctor trusts the patient to follow the treatment plan. Without this kind of trust there is no doctor-patient relationship.

Communication is as much about listening as it is about talking. Both the patient and doctor must listen attentively to one another. If you are unsure about what the doctor told you, repeat it back, and ask if you are correct. Ask for a clearer explanation if you need it. In a good relationship, the doctor will do the same for you. You have the right to a clear explanation so that you can manage your health. The doctor has a right to have clear communication from you in order to help you manage your illness. (More about communicating with your doctor in Question 31.)

If you are unsure about what the doctor told you, repeat it back, and ask if you are correct.

PART TWO

Stages of Grieving

Did I cause my disease?

If I'm never going to get better,
why bother trying?

How can I manage depression?

More . . .

7. Why me?

Why me? Why now? There is so much I haven't done yet. Is this the beginning of the end? I'm not ready. What did I do to deserve this disease? I must be a bad person. This must be a punishment. Did I cause this disease? If only I had exercised more, eaten better, stopped stressing, etc. Will I lose my independence? My mind? My life? My hopes and dreams?

Why not me? Why not now? Are there things I can still do? Am I still breathing and thinking and reading? Is anyone ever ready to have a chronic illness? Can all this wondering, worrying, and blaming change what's happening right this very second?

People get sick, and people die. We all know that. We just have a hard time believing it will happen to us. Every second we spend trying to answer these questions is a second we have lost in the present moment. Every ounce of energy we use pondering these questions is an ounce of energy we could have used to learn to manage our disease. Yesterday is a cancelled check. Tomorrow is a promissory note. Today (and this minute) is cash in hand. Spend it wisely.

8. Did I cause my disease?

It's my fault. If it's not my fault it has to be somebody's. Maybe it's genetic. You rack your brains searching for a family member who gave you the faulty genes. Are you just plain defective? Did your parents do drugs or drink or smoke? Were they exposed to radiation or toxic chemicals?

Maybe it's something around you: pollution, genetically modified crops, pesticides, drinking water, fluoride, vaccinations, radiation, or the hole in the ozone layer.

You name it, you can blame it. There has to be a reason, and you won't rest until you find it.

People will even try to blame you for your own illness. They can't make sense out of why this happened to you. (You can't make sense of it either.) If chronic illness, or acute illness for that matter, happens randomly, then everyone is at risk. That's terrifying! The immediate reaction is to lay blame somewhere, usually on the victim. So we are twice cursed. Blaming the victim is nothing new. The Old Testament story of Job is a perfect example. Job lost everything—possessions, family, livestock, and his health. Three friends came to console him. After sitting silently with Job for 1 week, they finally spoke. What did they say? Job must have done something to incur God's wrath!

In the New Testament, there is the story of the man born blind. People ask Jesus who sinned: the man or his parents? Someone had to bear the blame for this man's blindness. In recent times, a fundamentalist minister went so far as to publicly blame the residents of New Orleans for the devastation brought about by hurricane Katrina, saying that they deserved it! People have always tried to explain the inexplicable, usually by blaming someone.

You will probably blame yourself, too. You will look back over your life and find all the times you should have taken better care of yourself. You will recall all the health warnings and information that you ever read or heard on the news or from another person. If you had only known that your behavior would bring you to this end, you would have made different choices. Fill in the blank, "I should have_____." There are as many answers as there are people who get sick.

Blame serves no useful purpose. When others blame the victim, they are not protected from what they fear most—becoming victims of illness themselves. Their self-righteousness does nothing to alleviate our suffering. Their judgments don't console. Blaming ourselves doesn't help, either. In fact, it is downright destructive. The time and energy you spend trying to figure out what you did wrong or berating yourself won't change the fact that you are sick. That time and energy could be directed toward creating the best life possible. If an honest examination of your past reveals that you could have made better choices, resolve to do that right now. Dwelling in that past, however, robs you of the present. Dwelling in the past keeps you hopeless and helpless. When you look at the past, learn from it, and decide to live in the present moment, you become an empowered patient.

9. Does my disease cause all my problems or do other things come into play?

When you have a chronic illness, many other things can make problems worse or cause new problems. Kate Lorig, developer of the Chronic Disease Self-Management Workshops, writes about the symptom cycle in *Living a Healthy Life with Chronic Conditions*. The disease, which is at the center, can cause a variety of other symptoms like depression, anxiety, fear, pain, fatigue, muscle tension, and poor breathing. Each of those symptoms can lead to others in the cycle. For example, constant pain may lead to anxiety and fear which in turn lead to muscle tension, which causes even more pain.

In order to manage your symptoms, it is helpful to realize that not all of the symptoms come directly from the disease. And any one of the symptoms can make the disease worse. As a person with a chronic illness, you are the only one who can identify what is going on with you and this symptom cycle. And to complicate matters even more, once you break the cycle, it will repair itself. It's your job to be aware and to take the steps necessary to break the cycle each time.

Poor nutrition is another problem. When you are sick, you are not as inclined to eat what is best for you. Instead, you may reach for the food that comforts you. You probably don't have a lot of energy to spend on food preparation, so prepared food that is loaded with blood pressure-raising sodium, refined carbohydrates, and **artery**-clogging fat may be the norm. Without good nutrition, your body has an even harder time coping with disease. Poor nutrition is likely to lead to obesity, making your body work harder to do even the simplest things. Lack of exercise leads to fatigue, more pain, muscle tension, and sleep problems, while also contributing to obesity.

Artery

Blood vessel carrying blood away from the heart to the body.

10. Is denial a bad thing?

Denial is a normal part of adjusting to the diagnosis of a chronic illness. In the denial stage, we feel numb. We feel as if we have been transported into some stranger's life or that we are strangers observing our own lives from outside. At first, denial is good. Denial protects us from thinking about the unthinkable. Denial gives us time to adjust, to come to terms with the diagnosis. Healthy people may perceive this period of denial as a flaw and judge us. Each person has to accept his own diagnosis in his own time and his own way.

The denial that says, "I don't have it; they are wrong," is a denial that can only last a few days or weeks at most. After that, denial takes subtle destructive forms.

Wanting a second opinion may be wise. Wanting a tenth opinion when the first nine doctors all agree could be denial (and pretty expensive denial at that). Not following a treatment regimen can be denial. We get tired of reminders of illness, and conveniently forgetting to take medication or self-manage our illness can be denial. Pushing yourself beyond your limits is another way of pretending your limitations do not exist. Denial may speak in the words, "What difference does it make anyway?"

Let denial be the short-term buffer it is meant to be, and then move on to learn to manage your disease.

Let denial be the short-term buffer it is meant to be, and then move on to learn to manage your disease. Accepting the fact that you have a chronic condition is not resignation and it is not giving in or giving up. Norman Cousins, a journalist who suffered from **ankylosing spondylitis**, said, "Never deny a diagnosis, but do deny the negative verdict that comes with it."

Ankylosing spondylitis

An autoimmune disease that affects the spine and causes the bones to fuse together.

11. Why am I so angry all the time?

You get angry, angrier than you have ever been. What are you supposed to do with this anger? You can turn the anger inward. But anger turned inward is depression. You get mad at yourself for being depressed and then get even more depressed. If you do a good enough job of suppressing anger, you'll end up feeling nothing—bad or good. Either you feel your feelings or you don't. There is no picking and choosing, no middle ground.

You can turn your anger outward. When you do that, you alienate the very people you need to be there for you. Who wants to be around an angry person? You don't even like being around yourself when you are angry. You end up alone. And once again, you get mad at yourself and end up more depressed.

You can get angry at your body parts. A lot of good that does! When you are angry at your body, you don't take care of yourself. Nobody wants to care for a traitor, not even you. And you get sicker.

You are frightened, confused, and frustrated. Your life is out of control. This wasn't supposed to happen. Not now. Not to you. It's over too soon. You didn't choose this journey. Of course you're angry. Any person in his right mind would be!

12. What can I do to manage my anger?

If you can't repress anger and you can't express it without alienating others, what are you supposed to do? Accept the fact that you are angry. Buried feelings don't die. This anger is part of you and you can't just cut it out and toss it away. Nothing changes until you accept where you are right now. Words are powerful tools for dealing with anger. Write about what you feel. Talk to a good friend or a counselor. Beat a pillow; yell out loud in the car or when you are alone. Sure, it sounds silly, but what do you have to lose by trying? What do you have to gain? Channel your anger into learning about your condition and managing it. Get involved, and work for a cure. Make a difference.

Journaling is an excellent way to examine, express, and begin to release anger. You don't need a fancy book for journaling, just a simple notebook, a pen, and some quiet time. Start with an open-ended statement like "I am angry because . . ."; "I feel angry when . . ."; or something similar. Don't worry about grammar, spelling, or punctuation. And don't judge yourself for what you are feeling. The only rule is to keep the pen moving. Try to write for 20 minutes each time. Each time you write, the difficult emotion of anger will lose some of its power. Difficult emotions have a half-life very much like radioactive substances. Each time you express the emotion it loses half its power until it is little more than a faint background noise.

In the meantime, try to be aware of anger, especially when you feel like you are going to erupt and do all kinds of damage to your relationships with others. The old adage to "count to 10" is good advice. If you do react inappropriately, apologize the second you realize what you have done. Most people will understand if you offer a prompt and sincere apology.

David J.'s comment:

I know I should probably exercise and eat better. But what's the use? I'm never going to get rid of this disease. If I am going to have to spend the rest of my life being miserable, I am going to do what I want. At least I can enjoy my chips, soda, and candy. They are the only pleasures I have left. And those medications? They won't cure me. They can cause all kinds of problems. It's no use. I am going to do just what I want to do. I deserve that much.

13. If I'm never going to get better, why should I bother trying?

For people who have suffered for years with a constellation of symptoms, a diagnosis, having a name for what is wrong, is something of a relief. For many, the initial relief quickly turns to despair. The illness model that most people know is one that fits acute illness. You get sick, you get treated, then you either recover or you die. The illness model for chronic illness is quite different. You get sick, you finally find out what is wrong, you get treated, and you stay sick but hopefully not as sick as you were without treatment. It's easy to give up.

While it is true that you will never be "normal" like you once were, or "normal" like healthy people you see, your life is not over unless you decide it is. Your body and your life may look like they are out of control. You feel hopeless, helpless, and powerless. It's time to let go of either/or thinking.

No one is either totally sick or totally well. Normally healthy people have times when they are sick. People with chronic illness have times when they feel normal. The degree of health that we experience is continuum, not one or the other. Regardless of where you are on that health continuum, you have the power to make a difference in your quality of life. You may never go back to your "old normal" so you have to create a "new normal." That new normal can be sitting around having a solo pity party, wishing things were different or it can be creating a new life where chronic illness is integrated into the whole but is not at the center. Once you make a conscious decision to accept the fact that you have chronic illness and it's not going away, you can turn your attention to being proactive in your medical care, attending to your health, and creating a new life.

14. What are the symptoms of depression?

Depression, like almost everything else that has to do with chronic illness, is complicated. Depression can have a physical cause. Depression can be the result of pain and fatigue, but depression can cause pain and fatigue as well, setting an endless cycle in motion. Depression may come as a result of your situation. Loss of work, identity, health, and self-esteem can lead to depression. The journey to acceptance in chronic illness is similar to the journey of grieving for someone you love—but that someone is you and you're not dead yet. You grieve for who you were and for lost hopes and dreams. A lot of the time you feel hopeless and helpless. Depression is a stage in the grieving process.

You might not even realize that you are depressed. In a chronic illness workshop, the participants were asked to list symptoms of depression: loss of interest in daily activities, changes in appetite, sleeping too much, not being able to sleep, crying, inability to control negative thoughts, concentration problems, lack of motivation, being short with others, etc. One participant at the workshop, a take-charge kind of woman, sat in her seat and said through quiet tears. "Oh my God," she said, "I just realized that I am depressed and have been for a long time." That was a turning point for her.

According to the Mayo Clinic, symptoms of depression include:

• Loss of interest in normal daily activities
• Feeling sad or down
• Feeling hopeless
• Crying spells for no apparent reason
• Problems sleeping
• Trouble focusing or concentrating
• Difficulty making decisions
• Unintentional weight gain or loss
• Irritability
• Restlessness
• Being easily annoyed
• Feeling fatigued or weak
• Feeling worthless
• Loss of interest in sex
• Thoughts of suicide or suicidal behavior
• Unexplained physical problems, such as back pain or headaches

Not everyone has every symptom. If you suspect that you are depressed, there's a good chance that you are.

15. How can I manage depression?

The depression that goes along with chronic illness is normal but only for a while. People with chronic illness go through the same stages of grieving as people do when someone they love dies. These stages include denial and isolation, anger, bargaining, depression, and finally acceptance. Not everyone experiences these stages in the same order. Each stage is usually revisited a number of times.

If your depression is the result of having chronic illness and is not **biochemical** in nature, there are some things you can try. Anything you do to stop thinking and start doing can be helpful. Whether it's cutting your toenails, watching a feel-good movie, or learning a new hobby, doing anything is better than sitting and obsessing about your illness and situation. Phone a friend, and resolve to really listen to the other person. Don't use the call as a chance to say out loud all the unpleasant things you have been thinking. Focus on the other person. Listen to your favorite music. Read a book. Take a walk. Plant a flower. Take a bath. Have a nice cup of tea. Think about things that bring you pleasure and pick one that you can do.

Biochemical

Relating to chemicals that are found in living organisms. Imbalances can cause disease and depression.

Change your thinking. What we think causes what we feel. First pay attention to what you are telling yourself. How much of it is negative, hopeless, and helpless? Write these thoughts down. Then write a positive statement that counters each thought. If you are thinking that you can't do "anything" anymore, the opposite might be "I can be a good listener to someone in need"; or "Now that I don't do ____ anymore, I have the time

Think about things that bring you pleasure and pick one that you can do.

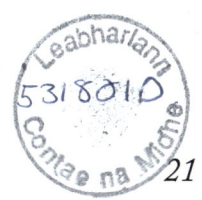

to learn _____, which I always wanted to do but never had the time before." Rehearse your new positive statements. Each time the negative statement creeps in, repeat the positive statement you have prepared.

16. How do I know when to see a professional about my depression?

Everyone has blue periods in their life. The fact that life has ups and downs is not news. But if you try strategies to lift your depression and if the symptoms of depression last for more than a few weeks, you will want to get professional help. Ask your doctor for a referral to a **psychologist** or **psychiatrist** so that you can be evaluated for depression. A good mental health professional will be able to determine whether your depression is biological, situational, or both, and guide you in choosing treatment options. And, as it is with chronic disease, the treatment of depression may involve some trial-and-error attempts on the part of patient and practitioner. For some people, there is a stigma attached to mental health counseling. They think it is only for those who are weak and crazy. Depression is just as real a disorder as insulin-dependent diabetes or a broken bone. You wouldn't try to treat those on your own, would you? It is the strong person, not the weak person, who has the courage to ask for help when needed. It is the sane person, not the crazy one, who makes a decision to relieve his own suffering.

Psychologist

A mental health professional who uses talk therapy and other techniques but does not prescribe medication.

Psychiatrist

A mental health professional who can prescribe medication to treat mental and emotional problems.

17. Why am I having trouble thinking and remembering?

Difficulty thinking and remembering can have several causes. There may be a biological cause for your cognitive problems that is based in the disease itself. The medications that you take to manage the disease or its symptoms may be the cause. Or the cause may be situational, brought on by the many stresses of living with a chronic medical condition. More than likely it is a combination of all three.

Autoimmune diseases can cause inflammation in the brain, affecting the ability to think clearly. **Neurological disorders** can skew the messages that travel from nerve to nerve. A quick search on the Internet turned up 371 diseases that can cause people to have problems with forgetfulness, trouble concentrating, confusion, and disorientation.

Medications that carry a warning that they may cause drowsiness and that you should avoid operating machinery after taking them can cause cognitive impairment, too. Pain medications, beta blockers, and steroids can all be culprits, among many others.

The constant stress of living with the uncertainty of chronic illness, pain, fatigue, and depression can all interfere with your ability to think clearly. If you add the challenges of loss of income, inability to pay for medical care, and changes in relationships resulting from chronic illness, is it any wonder that you have a hard time concentrating?

18. Why don't my prayers work?

Whether or not people profess faith in God or follow a spiritual path, they find themselves trying to bargain their way out of desperate situations. The old adage, "There are no atheists in foxholes" could easily apply to chronic illness. One of the stages of grieving—and remember we are grieving for our own losses—is bargaining. Whether it is bargaining with God as we know God or bargaining with something as vague as the cosmos, people will try to bargain their way out of

Autoimmune disease
Any disease in which a person's immune system cannot tell the difference between viruses, bacteria, or parasites and the healthy self.

Neurological disorders
Problems affecting the nervous system.

the illness. The process starts when the patient looks back at his or her life and decides that his less-than-perfect lifestyle or attitude is the cause of the sickness. The next step is making promises about future behavior in return for relief from the sickness. Bargaining sounds something like this, "If I get better (or You make me better) I promise I will (eat more vegetables, be nice to my neighbor, be a pleasant person, etc.). Bargaining makes some faulty assumptions. The first is that we did something to deserve our illness. The second is that our illness was inflicted on us as some kind of religious or cosmic punishment. The third is that whoever we are bargaining with will remove our sickness the same way that it was "given" it to us.

Instead of spending your energy figuring out what constitutes an enticing offer, put your energy into something you know will pay off and make a plan to manage your disease.

Whether or not you contributed to your illness is only important in that you have learned to change your behavior. What happened has happened, and nothing can change it. While prayer and meditation can be very helpful in managing chronic illness, playing "Let's Make a Deal" is not. Fortunately, the bargaining stage usually doesn't last very long. Instead of spending your energy figuring out what constitutes an enticing offer, put your energy into something you know will pay off and make a plan to manage your disease.

PART THREE

Impact of Chronic Illness on Social Relationships

Why do I feel so isolated?

How can I make other people understand what I am going through?

Should I tell people about my condition?

More . . .

Natasha M.'s comment:

I never go out anymore. How can I? I never know when I will have to get to a bathroom really fast! It's so embarrassing. I have to be so careful about what I eat. People are always telling me to try just a little of this or that, one slip won't hurt. They are so wrong. I don't want to offend anybody, but I don't want to make my disease the topic of conversation. Most of the time, I am too tired to entertain. And even when I am around people, I have nothing much to talk about. I don't work. I don't go out except to the doctor. I just don't fit anymore.

19. Why do I feel so isolated?

Chronic illness isolates us. The rest of the world seems to be going on about their business while you are left on the outside looking in, with your disease your only companion. Society has rituals for dealing with illness. If you are just a little sick, people will wish you well. If you are medium-sick people may even offer to help you out. If you are extremely sick, they will send flowers and cards, offer to go shopping for you, or bring you cooked meals. All of these rituals are based on the model of acute illness; that is, you get sick, then you get treated, then you get better (or die). When you are first diagnosed with chronic illness, people may experience all of these things. Then they expect you to get better. When you don't get better, most people feel like they have "done their duty" for you and go on about their lives. You take your disease by the hand and slink off into the shadows.

Some people will avoid you because you represent something terrifying—their own frailty and their own mortality. If you got this disease, that means they can get an incurable disease too! Let's face it, we all think we're invincible most of the time. When you have to look in the eyes of someone who has cancer, diabetes, **epilepsy**, or **multiple sclerosis**, you can't continue to

Epilepsy

A neurological condition that sometimes produces brief disturbances (seizures) in the normal electrical functions of the brain.

Multiple sclerosis

An autoimmune disease that affects the myelin sheath (covering) of the nerve pathways and disrupts communication to the muscles and other parts of the body.

ignore the fact that sooner or later everyone dies, and some of us get sick a long time before that. You now represent sickness, vulnerability, loss of control, and death. Others might avoid you in order to avoid the reality you represent. But you don't get to avoid that reality. You live with it every day.

Others feel awkward around sick people. They don't know what to say. "Get well soon" doesn't seem right when there is no cure in sight. They are afraid that if they talk about their own lives and activities, then you will feel worse because you can't do those things anymore. Over and over the discussion seems to come back to your illness or to an uncomfortable silence. In time, you and the others have less and less in common. Friendships and relationships falter and sometimes fail altogether.

You may contribute to your own isolation, whether you realize it or not. Healthy people take the greeting, "Hi, how are you?" to be nothing more than that, a passing greeting. But you feel isolated. You want to tell someone how you really feel. And you do tell them. You get nauseous from the drugs. Your bones and joints ache and creak. The doctor is sending you for a **CT scan, magnetic resonance imaging (MRI)**, or is putting cameras in your body where no cameras ought to go! Who wants to listen to that? Nobody I know!

As acquaintances fall by the wayside, you rely more and more on partners and close family to relieve your isolation. It's easy to forget that your loved ones feel as helpless as you do. They want desperately to do something to help you. When you spend all of your time trying to get them to understand how you feel by endlessly explaining your symptoms, they feel even more helpless and frustrated. Is it any wonder you feel isolated?

CT scan

A non-invasive medical test. CT imaging combines special X-ray equipment with sophisticated computers to produce multiple images of the inside of the body. These cross-sectional images of the area being studied can then be examined on a computer monitor or printed.

Magnetic resonance imaging (MRI)

A non-invasive medical test. MRI uses a powerful magnetic field, radio frequency pulses, and a computer to produce detailed pictures of organs, soft tissues, bone, and virtually all other internal body structures.

27

You may turn down invitations because you don't know how you will feel. If you say yes on Tuesday for a Thursday event, you may crash before then. You are afraid to say yes and then cancel. You worry about what people will think of you. Perhaps your disease manifests itself in some obvious way like seizures or having to run to the bathroom unexpectedly. You don't want to face the embarrassment so you don't go out. Or your pain and fatigue make the mere idea of socializing overwhelming.

But there is another kind of isolation. You know it by this intense, stabbing feeling of aloneness. You don't fit anymore. You are a stranger in the land of the healthy. Life is going on, but your life is on hold. You wish just one person could really be there with you, understand your experience, and feel your pain. And no matter how nice they are, the healthy folks just don't get what it is like to be you. You feel cut off, isolated, terribly alone. Isolation leads to depression, which in turn leads to more isolation.

20. What can I do about isolation?

First, accept the fact that some people can't handle being around people who are sick. You can't control them or what they do, but you can control your reactions. You can choose to obsess about these people or you can choose to put your limited energy somewhere more productive.

Second, be aware of what comes out of your mouth. What you say is a reflection of what you are thinking. Can you go through an hour with someone and not mention your condition? How about a day? Awareness of what you are doing is the first step to change.

Third, find a support group. Support groups and how to find them are dealt with in Question 93. Contacting a foundation that focuses on your disease is a good way to start.

Fourth, recognize that although chronic illness takes a toll on you, it also affects those who love you. Listen to your loved ones. Encourage them to share their own struggles with your disease. You are less alone than you imagine.

You are less alone than you imagine.

Finally, reach out to others. Write thoughtful letters, send cards, do little, unexpected nice things for people for no apparent reason. There are so many other people who are isolated just like you. "Reach out and touch someone" is more than an advertising slogan.

21. Why do I feel like a stranger to myself and others?

Chronic illness robs us of our identity, hopes, and dreams. Once the diagnosis is pronounced we will never be the same again. Susan Sontag, in her book *Illness as Metaphor*, writes that when we are diagnosed we become citizens of the land of the sick, only visiting the land of the well on a passport. We are foreigners in their world.

Once upon a time you identified yourself by your work, relationships, and hobbies; now you identify yourself as having "The Disease." The Disease is the last thing on your mind when you fall asleep and the first thing on your mind when you wake up in the morning. Your hopes and dreams for the future are dashed. Your identity is gone. Without that identity, you are a stranger to yourself and to the people with whom you had relationships. You feel like a stranger because you have indeed become a stranger.

But the loss of identity gives us an opportunity to create a new identity, a new normal. Stripped of our identity as human "doings" we can learn to be human "beings."

Peter J.'s comment:

I just don't know how to make my family "get it." I give them books. I show them things on the Internet. I tell them how I feel. They don't seem to care. I asked my sister to go with me to my doctor's appointment. She sat in the waiting room. Maybe if she came in with me, she would realize what this disease does. I asked her to come to the support group with me. Maybe if she hears what all of us are going through, she will understand. I keep trying but nothing works. What can I do?

22. How can I make other people understand what I am going through?

There is a scene in the movie *Gone with the Wind* where Melanie is about to give birth just as the Yankee troops are attacking Atlanta. Scarlett O'Hara and Prissy, the young slave girl, are her only attendants. Prissy goes to get a knife to put under the bed because, "Mama says it cuts the pain in half." Wouldn't it be nice if that worked? When we are suffering the effects of chronic illness—pain, fatigue, fear, loss of control, anger, despair—we want to cut the physical and emotional pain in half. We think that if the people around us could just understand what we are going through, our suffering would somehow be reduced. Like the knife under the bed, it doesn't work.

While it may be comforting to have people empathize with you and stand by your side, ultimately each of us has to go through the experience alone inside ourselves.

This is a very difficult life lesson. It's a lesson I learned while delivering my first child. I read all the books, attended the childbirth classes with my husband, made sure my doctors knew what my wishes were, and even visited the maternity ward ahead of my due date. I had my coach and my team, and everything would be just fine. The labor was 22 very long hours! During that time I realized that no matter who was with me, the contractions were mine, and the pushing was mine. People could be around me to do their part and to remind me what my part was, but the experience was mine alone.

Each person's experience of chronic illness is unique to that person. And as in childbirth, we may have helpers, but ultimately we go through the experience alone inside ourselves. Patients in support groups frequently complain that their healthy partners and others, "Just don't get it. They don't understand." They don't. They really can't. They are not experiencing what the patient is experiencing. You can get so hung up on making others understand that they get tired of your explanations and endless description of symptoms. The Disease with a capital "D," and your efforts to make others understand, becomes your only topic for conversation. When that happens, not only do the others not understand, they don't even want to because you have been driving them crazy. You drive them away.

The central question here is why do you need them to understand? Once you realize that their understanding will not change your situation, you can stop focusing on them and turn your attention to your own self-management. Part of that self-management means asking for appropriate help and support when you need it but not expecting others to be able to walk in your shoes.

23. How does chronic illness affect intimacy?

When one partner has a chronic illness, incredible stress can be put on intimate relationships. Some statistics place the rate of divorce at 75% when one partner is chronically ill! There are many reasons for these statistics, and lack of physical intimacy is certainly one of them.

The illness itself and the side effects of medications can cause physical changes in your body that leave you feeling unattractive and undesirable. Extreme changes in weight, deformities, scarring from surgeries and procedures, hair loss, and other changes leave you wondering why anyone would even want to be intimate with you. If you don't like yourself, why would anyone else like you? Rather than risk rejection, you avoid the issue altogether. When you do that, you are making a decision for your partner. You have no right to do that. The result is that your partner feels rejected, and the relationship begins to deteriorate. Good communication skills are essential for partners to sustain a relationship in the face of chronic illness. If those skills are not already in place, go see a counselor who can teach both of you how to make your feelings and needs made known in healthy ways.

Good communication skills are essential for partners to sustain a relationship in the face of chronic illness.

The constant pain and fatigue that often accompany chronic conditions are not conducive to intimacy, especially if intimacy is defined as an athletic sexual event rather than an emotional one. Redefining your perception of intimacy as close human contact, physically or emotionally, rather than a physical act, changes both partners' expectations. The sick partner may long to be held, cuddled, or kissed gently but is afraid to make any overtures out of fear that the healthy partner will take these overtures as a signal that more is to come.

Of course, the healthy partner may be very happy to hug and cuddle if that's what comforts the sick partner. But no one will know what the other is thinking or what the other needs without those needs being spoken.

The use of "I" messages is especially important here. "I would like to snuggle with you for a while. I feel good when we do that. I am afraid that you will think I want more, and right now, I'm just not up to that. Are you OK with this?" Again, a visit or two to a good mental health counselor can work wonders for communication skills that will preserve the relationship.

Pain can be a particularly difficult obstacle to physical intimacy. If this is a problem for you, talk to your doctor. He or she may have suggestions. You are not the first person to experience intimacy problems related to your chronic condition, and you won't be the last. You deserve to have as full a life as you can. Why not ask for the help you need? If your doctor is unable to help you, consult a physical therapist. You will be amazed at what you learn. A woman who had both hips replaced when she was only 22 (she's now in her late 40s) learned that having sex in the bathtub works best for her, as the water minimizes weight!

24. Should I tell people about my condition?

Chronic illness can be visible or invisible. You can't hide the deformities that come with **rheumatoid arthritis** or the rashes that accompany **psoriasis**. But many chronic illnesses are not apparent to the casual observer. If you have invisible chronic illness, you are faced with the "to tell or not to tell" dilemma. The decision of whether or not to disclose has to be taken on a situation-by-situation basis.

Rheumatoid arthritis

An autoimmune disease in which the immune system attacks and destroys the joints.

Psoriasis

Chronic, autoimmune disease that appears on the skin. It occurs when the immune system sends out faulty signals that speed up the growth cycle of skin cells.

33

Of course, you will want to tell those people who are close to you like spouses, parents, siblings, and adult children. If you have young children, you will want to be more guarded, giving them information on a need-to-know basis. Children need to be children and not your confidant, primary caregiver, or a substitute for a support network. They do need to know, however, that there are times when you may not be able to keep up with what other parents are doing. In all your relationships remember that you are more than your illness. Don't let your condition become the center of your relationships.

One of the frustrating things about chronic illness is unpredictability. You make plans for next week, only to find that on the day of the event, you are just too tired or sick to follow through. If your friends and acquaintances don't know about your condition, they will probably lose patience with you sooner or later. If they know about your illness, there is a better chance that they will understand. Some people will become overprotective. They will remind you to rest, eat, or whatever, leaving you feeling like you are a helpless child. Some people, however, won't get it. Convincing them is not worth your limited energy. The decision to disclose is very personal. Remember that you can't control how others will react or how they will treat you. The only reactions that you can control are yours.

Casual acquaintances really don't need to know about your health. You don't tell them how much money is in your bank account, or how often you floss your teeth, or about your crazy Uncle Joe. If you find yourself telling relative strangers about your illness, you might want to think about the possibility that you are letting the illness define who you are. When mere acquaintances ask how you are doing, they are being polite and not asking for a laundry list of your symptoms and ailments or a graphic description of your latest medical procedure.

Chronic illness in the workplace is a tricky issue. Employers and bosses, just like anyone else, will have preconceived notions about your illness. If you are doing your job and don't need special accommodations, there is no good reason to disclose your illness in the workplace. Even if you have a great relationship with your co-workers, most of them are not close friends or family and do not need to know the details of your physical condition. If you do need special accommodations, then disclose to only those people who need to know. Even though you are supposed to be protected under the Americans with Disabilities Act, the sad truth is, if your illness is perceived as a burden to your employer they will find a way to get rid of you. The best advice here is to be guarded when it comes to disclosing in the workplace.

PART FOUR

Chronic Illness and the Law

What rights do I have under the Americans with
Disabilities Act?

What is the Family Medical Leave Act,
and how does it affect me?

How can I be sure that my wishes will
be honored if I am unable to make medical
decisions for myself?

More . . .

Joy M.'s comment:

My disease makes me very sensitive to sunlight and fluo-rescent light. The light makes my disease flare. Of course, we have fluorescent lights in the office. There are about 10 of us working in cubicles in this single room. I can't control the light. I asked my boss to put filters on the lights, and she refused. She said it was too expensive. She even laughed at me because she didn't believe that the lights could make me sick. This is discrimination! Isn't there a law about this? What about the ADA, doesn't it say that employers have to make reasonable accommodations for people who need it? Maybe I should get a lawyer!

25. What rights do I have under the Americans with Disabilities Act?

Some chronic illnesses are disabling. According to the Council for Disability Rights:

Forty-three million Americans have physical or mental dis-abilities. Too often they are excluded from the mainstream of American life by attitudes and inaccessible environments. Sixty-seven percent of all people with disabilities are unem-ployed, even among college graduates. The ADA benefits all of us. Each of us has a 20% chance of becoming a person with a disability and a 50% chance of having a family member with a disability.

The Americans with Disabilities Act (ADA) recog-nized that the disabled are often discriminated against. The ADA defines the rights of the disabled much like the Civil Rights Act of 1964 addressed racial discrimi-nation. But the ADA is often misunderstood.

The ADA covers people with disabilities that substan-tially limit one or more major life functions (eating, breathing, caring for oneself, working, walking, etc.). When it comes to employment, only companies with more than 15 employees are required to comply. If you ask for accommodations and the employer can prove that it is an undue hardship, the employer does not have to comply. And an employer does not have to provide reasonable accommodations unless the employee asks for them.

Employers are not allowed to ask job applicants about disabilities. Employers are allowed to ask if the applicant can perform the duties of a job. Medical examinations can only be required if they are job related, consistent with the employer's business needs, and required of all employees entering similar jobs. Drug testing is permitted. Any medical information obtained by the employer must be kept confidential. Employers who hire disabled people may be eligible for a small business tax credit. The ADA also covers accessibility to public transportation, to existing buildings and new construction in public accommodations, as well as communication media.

Be advised that no matter how well-crafted and no matter how well-intentioned this act is, people find ways to circumvent it and discriminate anyway. The law is good. It's just not foolproof. If employers want to get rid of you because of a disability or a request for reasonable accommodation, they will find another way. Proving discrimination may be difficult. If you decide to do that, be sure you understand the law and be certain that your case is well documented.

26. What is the Family Medical Leave Act (FMLA), and how does it affect me?

If you have a chronic illness and are still able to work, there's a good chance that between your illness and the number of medical appointments required, you will use up any sick or paid time off before you make it through half a year. Once you use up your paid time off, you might be able to invoke the Family Medical Leave Act (FMLA). Here are some things you should know.

FMLA applies to all public agencies, including state, local, and federal employers, local education agencies (schools), and private-sector employers who employed 50 or more employees in 20 or more workweeks in the current or preceding calendar year, including joint employers and successors of covered employers. If you work for a small business with a handful of employees, you are not covered.

To be eligible for FMLA benefits, an employee must:

- Work for a covered employer
- Have worked for the employer for a total of 12 months
- Have worked at least 1,250 hours over the previous 12 months
- Work at a location in the United States or in any territory or possession of the United States where at least 50 employees are employed by the employer within 75 miles.

A covered employer must grant an eligible employee up to a total of 12 workweeks of unpaid leave during any 12-month period for one or more of the following reasons:

- For the birth and care of a newborn child of the employee
- For placement with the employee of a son or daughter for adoption or foster care
- To care for a spouse, son, daughter, or parent with a serious health condition

- To take medical leave when the employee is unable to work because of a serious health condition
- For qualifying exigencies arising out of the fact that the employee's spouse, son, daughter, or parent is on active duty or call to active duty

Your employer is required to maintain your group health insurance during FMLA. You are required to make whatever contribution to that insurance that you were making prior to taking leave. When you return to work, you have rights to job restoration. Upon return from FMLA leave, an employee must be restored to the employee's original job, or to an equivalent job with equivalent pay, benefits, and other terms and conditions of employment. FMLA is not paid leave.

Your employer is required to maintain your group health insurance during FMLA.

Just as with invoking the ADA, good judgment and caution should be used when deciding to use FLMA. When in doubt consult an attorney who specializes in labor law.

27. What do I have to do in order to get Social Security Disability Insurance (SSDI) payments?

Many people have misconceptions about SSDI. In order to qualify, you must have paid in enough credits to Social Security. This is because SSDI is an insurance policy underwritten by the U.S. government. If you haven't paid enough credits, you cannot qualify for this benefit. The value of credits changes from year to year and exceptions are made for younger people who have not worked long enough to accumulate enough credits. Contact the Social Security Administration to see if you might qualify. SSDI is not your own money, even though you paid into the system. The money workers are paying right now pays for the benefits for people who are receiving SSDI right now.

Social Security has some very specific criteria for determining disability. The following is taken from their Web site:

The definition of disability under Social Security is different than other programs. Social Security pays only for total disability. No benefits are payable for partial disability or for short-term disability.

"Disability" under Social Security is based on your inability to work. We consider you disabled under Social Security rules if:

- You cannot do work that you did before.
- We decide that you cannot adjust to other work because of your medical condition(s).
- Your disability has lasted or is expected to last for at least 1 year or to result in death.

This is a strict definition of disability. Social Security program rules assume that working families have access to other resources to provide support during periods of short-term disabilities, including workers' compensation, insurance, savings, and investments. Before applying for these benefits you should check to see if you have enough credits, talk with all of your doctors, and seriously consider consulting an attorney who specializes in Social Security.

If approved, your payments cannot start until you have been disabled for at least 5 full months. Generally, your disability benefits will continue as long as your medical condition has not improved and you cannot work.

Benefits will not necessarily continue indefinitely. Because of advances in medical science and rehabilitation techniques, many people with disabilities recover from serious accidents and illnesses. Your case will be reviewed at regular intervals to make sure you are still disabled. You are responsible for telling the Social Security Administration if your medical condition improves, if there is any change in your ability to work, or if you return to work. Depending on the amount of your payments, you may even have to pay income tax on them. You will not be eligible to enroll in Medicare until you have received benefits for 2 full years.

28. What is HIPAA?

HIPAA stands for the Health Insurance Portability and Accountability Act. The law has many provisions about fraud and finances and such, but the Privacy Rule is particularly relevant when dealing with chronic illness. The HIPAA Privacy Rule creates national standards to protect individuals' medical records and other personal health information. You have the right to control the disclosure of your personal health information including:

- Advance consent for most disclosures of health information
- The right of individuals to see a copy of their health records
- The right to request correction of inaccurate health records
- The right to obtain documentation of disclosures of their health information
- The right to an explanation of their privacy rights and how their information may be used or disclosed

These are your *rights*. Read them again. The days of your medical records being kept from you are over. If you see something that is wrong, you can request that it be corrected. Note that you have a right to see your health records. If you want a copy, you might be charged a nominal fee. You will find that it is worth the trouble.

HIPAA also safeguards your personal medical information. In the vast majority of cases, a patient's health care information can only be used for such purposes as treatment and payment. Employers cannot obtain your personal information for the purpose of hiring, firing, or determining promotions without your consent. Insurance companies cannot use your personal health information for the purpose of underwriting products like life insurance. You can learn more about HIPAA on the U.S. Department of Health and Human Services Web site (http://www.hhs.gov/ocr/privacy/index.html).

29. How can I be sure that my wishes will be honored if I am unable to make medical decisions for myself?

No one wants to think or talk about critical care or end-of-life issues. You may have mentioned your opinions about what you would like to happen if you are not able to make your wishes known to medical providers, but that is not enough to make sure your wishes are carried out. Your loved ones may have opinions that are different from yours. Your loved ones may interpret what you said very differently. Take time to think about what you want. Do you want every effort made to keep you alive, no matter what that is? Do you want nutrition and hydration but not a ventilator? Discuss your wishes with your doctor. Put them in writing and have it witnessed. Your local hospital will probably

Discuss your wishes with your doctor.

have a blank form that you can use. Don't put the copy away in your safe deposit box! If you can't speak for yourself, you certainly can't get into your safe deposit box to get this document. Give copies to all of your doctors, and have them placed in your chart. Explain your wishes to your doctors as well. Give copies to the family members who will most likely be charged with making sure this document is honored.

End-of-life issues are not the only ones with which you should be concerned. You may be temporarily incapacitated and not able to make decisions for yourself. In that case, you need a health care proxy or surrogate. It might be a family member. But remember, a family member will be influenced by his or her own emotions. A trusted and objective friend might be a better choice. You are the only person who knows. Again, your local hospital is a good resource for further information.

Review these documents at least once a year. Your changing health, changing relationships, and your own changing attitudes make this review a necessity. Aging with Dignity/Five Wishes and Hospice both have excellent materials to help you make decisions and create these documents. You will find contact information for these groups in the Appendix.

30. What should I know about my medical records?

Your medical records are extremely important. They provide a history of your health and your chronic illness. If new symptoms develop, these records will be helpful in the detective work that leads to an accurate diagnosis.

Your medical records are yours. You have a right to have a copy. It is legal for your provider to charge a nominal fee for making copies. You are less likely to get charged if you ask for copies of your most recent tests and such at the end of each visit. You also have a right to check the medical records for accuracy. This is especially important if you apply for any kind of disability. One sentence taken out of context can destroy your case.

All of your providers should have copies of all your records. It is your job as a patient to make sure this happens. Either hand-deliver a copy to your other providers or ask that these records be faxed to them. You want the best care possible, and that just won't happen if the right hand does not know what the left hand is doing.

PART FIVE

Medical Providers and Medical Organizations

How can I get my doctors to talk to one another about my medical care?

Why do I have to see doctors so often?

Can I fire my doctor? Can my doctor fire me?

How can I challenge decisions made by my insurance company?

More . . .

31. How can I get my doctor to listen to me and take me seriously?

This is by far the biggest complaint patients seem to have about doctors. Like everything else related to chronic illness, this problem has no simple answer. There are things you can do to improve the situation, however. Granted, doctors are usually very busy. Constraints put on them as a result of managed care might mean that they can't spend a lot of time with each patient. You can't change the system, and you can't change your doctor. That's sad, but it is reality. Doctors and patients rarely speak the same "language." What you can do is learn how the doctor likes to receive information and then, if necessary, change the way in which you communicate.

Doctors and patients rarely speak the same "language."

Often, patients have not prepared to maximize the time they have with the doctor. When they get into the exam room, they are already flustered, forget the most important things, and give ambiguous answers. The doctor has a hard time understanding. Instead of giving a clear picture of what they are experiencing, patients often give vague answers and hope that the doctor will ask questions to draw the information out of them. The following suggestions should make a difference in your doctor-patient relationship.

Come to your appointment prepared. Bring a written list of all prescriptions, medications, over-the-counter medications, vitamins, herbs, and supplements that you are taking. Include the name, dose, and frequency with which you take each. Have a copy for you and one for the doctor. This saves time and eliminates the possibility that your medications may not be entered correctly in your records. It is absolutely critical that you tell the doctor about everything you are taking. Some supplements work against certain medications you may be taking.

Others amplify the effects of your medication in undesirable ways. Still others can actually increase disease activity. You can't expect your doctor to be of much help if you hide this kind of critical information.

Learn to describe your symptoms clearly and in terms that will help your doctor help you. A symptom journal is an excellent way for you to track the information. Get a notebook, and record in it the following things: What is the symptom? When did it start? How often do you experience this symptom? What relieves the symptom? What makes it worse? How long does the symptom last? On a scale of 1 to 10 where 10 is the worst, how severe is the symptom? Does this symptom interfere with your ability to perform activities of daily living? If so, how? Make a short list of descriptive words regarding the symptom. Let's look at two hypothetical patients and their discussions with their doctors.

Patient 1

Doctor: *Good morning. How are you doing today?*
Patient: *Oh, I'm just kind of blah.*
Doctor: *What's the problem?*
Patient: *I feel achy.*
Doctor: *Where?*
Patient: *Well, it kind of moves around.*
Doctor: *Where do you feel it most often?*
Patient: *Hard to say.*
Doctor: *Can you describe the ache?*
Patient: *It's just sort of, you know, an ache. You have to give me something to make it go away.*

Patient 2

Doctor: *Good morning. How are you doing today?*
Patient: *Not too bad, but I am troubled by these aches and pains in my joints.*

Doctor: *Go on.*

Patient: *Every morning when I wake up, I am so sore and stiff that it takes me about 2 hours to get moving. After I have a long, hot shower I start to feel a little better.*

Doctor: *Which joints bother you the most?*

Patient: *The little joints in my hands, my wrists, and my feet and ankles.*

Doctor: *Let me take a look at them.*

Which patient do you think will be taken seriously, listened to, and have his or her needs addressed?

32. How can I get my doctors to talk with one another about my medical care?

You are the one person who knows what each doctor is doing. You are the one person who sees them all. And you are the one person who can make sure that all your medical providers are on the same page. Of course, there will be times when two of your doctors will consult with each other about your case, but this is not the norm. You can improve the overall quality of your care by taking on this responsibility.

Make sure all of your medical care providers have a current list of your medications, vitamins, supplements, and over-the-counter medications. Include the dose and how often you take each one. If you use one pharmacy, you are more likely to have the pharmacist notice if two medications have bad interactions. If all your doctors know what you are taking, you have an even better chance of avoiding problems.

Give copies of all your medical tests to all of your medical providers. Your lab is not going to fax your results to a long list of doctors. You doctors are not going to send your results to one another. When you see the doctor who ordered the tests, ask for a copy. These are your tests, you paid for them, and you have a right to have a copy of them. Then you can mail, fax, or hand-deliver those results to the rest of your doctors. They will become part of your chart and may provide clues about other problems.

The ultimate responsibility for the coordination of your medical care rests with you!

Samantha H.'s comment:

All of a sudden, I got this blinding headache. I have been through a lot but never felt anything so bad, so painful. I had trouble seeing. My doctor gave me a referral to a neurologist. The receptionist told me there was a 6-month wait. Six months! I couldn't live like this for 6 months! I explained what I was going through and begged her to call me if she had a cancellation or maybe ask the doctor to see me at the end of the day. She clearly didn't get it. The pain got worse. I called again. Finally, I called the doctor's service after hours. They paged the doctor. He called. After we talked he told me to go straight to the emergency room where he would meet me. It's a darned good thing too because I had an **aneurysm** *in my brain. They did surgery that night. And I am still alive to tell the tale!*

Aneurysm

Fluid-filled sac in the wall of a blood vessel that can weaken the wall and cause it to rupture.

33. How can I get past the staff at the front desk and make my concerns known to my doctor?

Not only do you have the frustrations of dealing with your chronic illness, you also have to deal with the front desk staff at your doctor's office. For some unknown reason, a lot of these people have forgotten

51

how to smile. Even worse, they have appointed themselves as protectors of the doctor. If your doctor has wonderful staff, you can skip this section. But sooner or later you will encounter the Gatekeepers. It's a good idea to be prepared.

The best thing you can do is be pleasant and very human with the Gatekeeper. Even though you may be stressed at having to be at the doctor's office, the Gatekeeper sees stressed people day in and day out and is somewhat immune to your distress. Smile, say hello, and say something nice. You are building the foundation of a relationship that you will need down the road. Use her name. Thank her. Pay her a compliment. You want her to remember you fondly when you call desperate to make an appointment or need the doctor to call you back.

You are building the foundation of a relationship that you will need down the road.

When you call, identify yourself by name and mention that you are a patient of doctor so-and-so. State your request clearly and concisely. Ask the person taking the message to repeat it back to you. A lot of information can be lost in translation! If you can, fax your request to the doctor. Follow up a little while later with a call asking if your fax was received, and instruct that person to give it to the doctor. This technique works very well. If you don't hear back within 24 hours, repeat the process.

If you have a true emergency, say so up front. If necessary, call 911 or go to the emergency room. If your medical need is pretty serious but not critical, you can use the technique of last resort—the after office hours call. Caution: Use this only in extreme circumstances or everyone, including the doctor, will be upset with you. Don't be the boy who cried wolf. When you call after hours, you get the answering service. They will then call your doctor who will decide how to respond.

Respect the doctor's time. Respect the Gatekeeper's job. But make sure you get the medical attention you need.

34. Why do I have to see so many doctors?

The human body is extremely complex. Each organ system is like an entire universe. Rarely does chronic illness affect just one part of the body. Think about your medical team in terms of football. Team Disease has many special players, each with their own unique offensive skills. You need a team, Team "Something-ologist" with specialists who know how to first defend against the attack and then go on the offensive themselves. If your entire team consisted of one quarterback you wouldn't stand a chance of winning. It is the same with chronic illness.

Your job in the game is to be the team manager. Once your "quarterback," or the doctor who is central to your care, tells you what team members you need, you go out and hire them. We'll discuss how to find good team members in Question 36. Over time you may add new members, replace members, or no longer have a need for others. A manager who has a winning team is always making adjustments.

Outside of assembling your team, you have another extremely important function. You are responsible for making sure all the members of the team are working from the same playbook. You are responsible for keeping all the team members informed about what the others are doing.

35. Why do I have to see doctors so often?

Healthy people usually see their doctors about once a year, a little more often as they reach advanced years. People with chronic illness may see their doctors as often as once a month! Why so often, if there is no hope of a cure? When you have a chronic illness, your disease might be stable for a long period of time or might become active in short order. Regular medical monitoring allows your doctor to catch changes early and take aggressive steps to bring problems under control. Even though you may be feeling better than usual or see no change in your condition, silent and symptomless damage might be going on. Your blood pressure could be elevated. Your liver might be experiencing stress and damage as a side effect of medications. **Cholesterol** could be building up in your blood vessels. Your kidneys could be experiencing early stages of disease. None of these things has symptoms in the early stages. Your regular visits to the doctor can catch these and other things. Damage can be halted or slowed.

So, why don't folks with chronic illness want to see doctors? When you have chronic illness, a visit to the doctor is full of emotional undercurrents. Every encounter with the medical system is a graphic reminder that you are sick. Then there is the fear factor. It's not that you are afraid of the doctor, but you may be afraid of what the results of your last test will show, what new treatment might be required, what scary test or treatment might be ordered next, and that there will be more bad news.

It's easy to become an ostrich, stick your head in the sand, and avoid the whole issue by missing or canceling appointments. But the fear is still there, and the disease is still there. Just because you don't know about a problem doesn't mean it ceases to exist. You want the best life possible. You want to avoid complications. You want to see your doctor as often as your doctor recommends.

Cholesterol

A waxy substance found naturally in the body and necessary for some bodily functions. Cholesterol is also found in foods. An excess of cholesterol can cause buildup in the arteries, leading to hardening of the arteries and disease.

36. *How can I find a good doctor?*

Choosing a doctor is difficult. Like everything else with chronic illness, there is no simple answer. Ask your principal doctor what specialists he or she recommends and why. Ask friends and family members. Check with the American Medical Association. Look at their credentials. But sadly, you can do all these things and still not be satisfied with the doctor.

The doctor may have great credentials and a spotless record but be rude, inattentive, fail to look at or listen to you, or even be burned out. A doctor with lesser credentials may be just as qualified and might even take the time to treat you like a human being. So before you set out on your quest for a doctor, do some thinking about what you need and want in your medical provider. Personally, I am not above popping into a doctor's waiting room to see how many patients are stacked up and listen to their comments. It doesn't take long to know if the patients believe the doctor is worth the wait.

Take all recommendations from friends and family with a grain of salt. The doctor-patient relationship is very personal. The doctor will know the intimate details of your health and life. And because you see your doctors so often, you will get to know them as people too. Just as we have preferences in choices of mates and friends, we all have preferences for personalities in our doctors. Aunt Matilda might swear by Dr. Jones, while your best friend Karen can't stand him.

Take time to think about your preferences and needs in a doctor. Do your homework. Try the doctor to see if you are a fit. Give the relationship a trial period. And remember to use good communication skills and be very professional about being a patient. It's your job!

Take time to think about your preferences and needs in a doctor.

55

37. Can I fire my doctor? Can my doctor fire me?

John came to a disease support group meeting full of questions. He was newly diagnosed, and the group was eager to answer his questions. At the end of the meeting, the group leader asked, "John, did you get what you needed out of this meeting?" He answered, "Oh I sure did. I learned that it is OK to fire my doctor. I just needed permission."

If the doctor-patient relationship isn't working you have three choices. You can silently endure the relationship and be miserable. You can work on the relationship and try to improve it. You can end the relationship. As a patient, you have the right to make any of these choices at any time. But remember that your doctor has the very same rights in the doctor-patient relationship. You don't have to go to that doctor. That doctor is not obligated to take you as a patient. Of course, if you find yourself going through doctors one after another, you will want to take a hard look at how you function in the doctor-patient relationship.

Anastasia R.'s comment:

Can you believe it? Just 6 months ago my insurance company told me that I have to get my medication from a "specialty pharmacy." After six phone calls, somebody finally found one in my city. I know it's a good idea to have all your prescriptions at the same place, so I transferred everything. Now, I get another notice that I have to change specialty pharmacies, and this one only does mail order. Are they crazy? The insurance won't approve a refill until I have only 7 days of medication left, but it takes 7 to 14 days for the medication to come! Are they just trying to kill me or something? They won't let me get a 90-day supply probably because the medication is so expensive they are afraid I will die and some pills will go to waste. And to top it all off, now I will have prescriptions being filled in more than one pharmacy. It's so frustrating, but they seem to hold all the cards.

38. How can I challenge decisions made by my insurance company?

Insurance companies have assumed a position of major power when it comes to getting medical care. Doctors are frustrated. Patients are frustrated. Insurance companies dictate which tests can be done and whether or not you can have surgery. If you are sick long enough, you will find yourself going head-to-head with your insurance company, if you are lucky enough to have insurance in the first place. If you are not proactive, you don't have a chance of winning.

If you disagree with your insurance company's edict, you have a right to appeal. Go to their Web site or call and find out what to do to file an appeal. It is critical to keep track of every phone call, every letter or fax, and every email. A small notebook dedicated to your encounters with the insurance people is an invaluable tool. Record the day and time of communication, the name of the person with whom you spoke, and the outcome of the conversation. Chances are that when you call the next time, a totally different person will tell you a totally different story. When you point out the discrepancy, they will ask, "Who told you that?" You want to be ready with the answer.

When you file a written appeal, explain the problem and offer acceptable solutions. For example, if you are being forced to get your medication through the mail, it takes 7 to 14 days for you to receive your medication, but the insurance will not authorize a refill until your medication is 75% used, then that is a problem. Simply point out the impact on your health. "I am at risk of going without my medication every single month." Offer solutions. In this case, solutions might be permission to refill the prescription when it is 50% used, getting a 90-day supply, or using a local pharmacy.

Although you may be told that an appeal takes 30 days, ask about rapid resolution. Always ask when a decision will be rendered and who you can call to follow up. If you are not happy with the information you receive from the representative, you can always say politely, "Clearly you do not have the authority or have the information I need. Please put your supervisor on the phone." Be insistent. There is always a supervisor present, regardless of what they tell you.

The people who answer the phone don't make the rules.

Remember, you or your employer pay dearly for this insurance. Health insurance companies are not charities that graciously offer to help you. You are paying for a service. The people who answer the phone don't make the rules. Try not to take your frustrations out on them personally, but be firm. When you are very sick it's hard to muster the strength to take on this struggle. Ask someone to help you. If necessary, give them limited power of attorney to deal with your insurance company.

PART SIX

Medication

Why don't I notice any positive changes when
I take my medications?

Why does my doctor keep changing my
medications and treatment plan? Is my doctor
experimenting on me?

How can I find help to pay for my medical
expenses and medications?

More . . .

39. Why should I keep taking these medications, especially when they have such dreadful side effects?

Everything that you put into your body has an effect on how your body functions. Put in saturated fat and trans fats and you can expect coronary artery disease. Put in alcohol and drugs and you can expect liver disease. Put in more calories than you burn and you can expect obesity and adult-onset diabetes. Smoke tobacco and you can expect a **chronic obstructive pulmonary disease (COPD)** and maybe even lung cancer. The majority of people don't seem to recoil from the side effects of our modern lifestyle. Have you ever heard someone say, "I don't want to inhale the formaldehyde that leeches into the air from my new sofa?" Of course not! But when we hear that we need to take medication, maybe for life, we zero in on the side effects and decide this medication is not for us!

Virtually all medications have potential side effects. Not taking medication has side effects, too. For example, treatment options for psoriasis might include methotrexate, cyclosporine, and acitretin, which may control the disease but present the risk of **end-organ toxicity**, the potential increased risk of infection and malignancies, as well as the long-term emergence of autoimmune responses. The issue here is risk versus benefit. Is the risk associated with this treatment worth the benefit that you can expect? Is there a way to monitor or minimize the potential side effects? Remember that the treatment of chronic illness is very different than the treatment of acute illness. In acute illness, the doctor calls the shots. In chronic illness, the patient and doctor collaborate in making treatment decisions. If you, as a patient, are going to make wise

Chronic obstructive pulmonary disease (COPD)
A disease of the lungs that hampers breathing and is often caused by smoking or exposure to inhaled chemicals.

End-organ toxicity
Problems that are caused by medication prescribed to treat another condition.

decisions, you have to do your homework and learn about the medication or treatment.

Once you have done your homework, have an honest discussion with your doctor. Come with a list of questions. If your doctor doesn't seem to have enough time to answer your questions in your scheduled appointment, ask for another appointment where you can have 15 minutes of uninterrupted attention so that you and the doctor can take some time to discuss your questions and concerns about various treatment options. Be prepared and honor that time. If your doctor is unwilling to have this discussion you can fire your doctor! On the other hand, it is important to respect the doctor's time. If you ask for a long discussion every week, your doctor may fire you! Just like the decision of whether or not to take a certain medication is about finding the balance between risk and benefit, your relationship with your doctor is about finding the balance between having the serious discussions you need versus monopolizing the doctor's time and energy.

In the end, you are the one who decides what goes into your body. Your decision must be an informed decision based on research, discussion, and weighing risk versus benefits. No one is going to do this for you. It's your illness, your treatment, and your life.

40. What is the difference between an allergic reaction to medication and a side effect?

It's easy to confuse allergic reactions to medication with side effects. Most medications have side effects. Nausea, headache, dizziness, and dry mouth are very common side effects. Side effects can be expected with the majority of medications that people take to manage chronic illness. You must assess for yourself the risk-versus-benefit ratio of medication. If the side effects are more troublesome to you than the disease, have an honest discussion with your doctor. There may be alternative medications that will work better for you without that level of side effects.

Allergic reactions are another matter. Allergic reactions usually appear shortly after you take the medication. They can range from mild to severe and even life-threatening. If you take a medication and break out in hives, that would be an allergic reaction. If you take medication and your eyes swell up and you have trouble breathing, that is an allergic reaction. For severe allergic reactions, don't wait; call 911. As soon as you receive medical attention, call the doctor who prescribed the medication. If this happens after office hours, you will get an answering service, and they will page the doctor. If the distinction between side effect and allergic reaction is not clear, have a discussion with your doctor.

41. Why don't I notice any changes when I take my medications?

If you have a headache you take aspirin, Tylenol, or ibuprofen. If you have a really bad headache like a migraine you might need a prescription. The medication enters your system and relieves the symptoms and sometimes the cause. If you have an infection you take antibiotics. Again, the medication enters your system and treats the cause, although in this case you have to take the antibiotic for a prescribed number of days in order for it to be truly effective.

Some medications prescribed for symptoms of chronic illness are designed to relieve the symptoms. Others are designed to address the source of the symptoms. These medications are typically taken for long periods of time, even for life. Their effectiveness builds up over time. So, unlike a headache remedy that may provide relief in short order, these drugs need to be taken regularly over a period of time before you see any noticeable improvement. The improvement may be so subtle at first that you hardly notice it. Likewise, if you stop the medication it may take some time before your symptoms return. The goal here is to prevent or minimize problems before they become troublesome, rather that treat them after they occur.

There are some medications that you should NEVER alter the dose or stop without your doctor's supervision. These include steroids, diabetes medication, antidepressants, blood pressure, and heart medications. Frequently, it is the patient who is most troubled by the possible risks of a treatment who is willing to gamble with the much higher risks of stopping or changing the dose willy-nilly. Deciding to play doctor, usually under the declaration of "I know my body better than anyone else," can very well mean that the morgue will know your body sooner rather than later.

42. Why does my doctor keep changing my medications and treatment plan? Is my doctor experimenting on me?

Patients often complain about how their doctors approach treatment. Doctors may change medications, increase or decrease doses, or add and subtract medications. Two patients with the same disease sitting in the doctor's waiting room may discover that their treatment plans are quite different. This ambiguity leaves patients wondering if the doctor knows what he or she is doing. Patients wonder if the doctor is guessing or, worse, experimenting. Nothing could be further from the truth.

No two patients experience the same chronic disease in exactly the same way. Because of that, there is no "cookie cutter" approach or single formula for treatment. There will certainly be similarities, but there will always be differences. Each person brings his or her own unique medical history and makeup to the disease. In addition, people who have one chronic condition will often have several different conditions that overlap. On top of all that confusion, your medical condition is not static—things are always changing. Since we have no cure for chronic illnesses yet, doctor and patient alike are saddled with the frustration of inadequate therapies. The bottom line is that the treatment plan must be individualized for each patient's unique medical circumstance. The treatment plan has to be adjusted with variations in disease activity and health.

One doctor likened the process to cooking. "We don't have a cookbook of recipes who telling us exactly what to use, how much, and how long to cook it. Instead we have a pretty good idea what can go in, but with any good cook, adjustments have to be made constantly until you get just the right combination."

43. How can I change the way I feel about taking medication?

Hardly anybody likes to take medication. The issue of risk versus benefit when it comes to virtually all medications was discussed earlier. Just because you have done your homework and had a serious discussion with your doctor about the risks compared with the benefits of your medications doesn't mean you will look forward to taking them. Every time you have to use medication you are reminded again that you are sick, that there is something wrong with you, and it's not going away. When patients "forget" to take medication, they may be avoiding the regular reminder of their condition. Not complying with the treatment regimen is a form of denial.

Is there anything you can do to feel better about medication and treatment? Yes! The first step is to change your relationship with the medication. Do you wince each time you use medication as you silently repeat the list of possible side effects in your mind? Not only is the act of taking medication a reminder of chronic illness, it also becomes a reminder of all the bad things that can result from the medication itself. If you are going to change your relationship with medication, then you have to start by changing your thinking.

Start by mentally listing the benefits of the medications each time you take a dose. When your thoughts go back to the negative, simply remind yourself that you are changing the way you think. This takes practice. You might even have to write down the list of benefits and read them each time you take a dose. Think or even say out loud, "I am taking this pill because it will do (this good thing) and this one because it will do (another good thing)."

Another way to change your thinking and therefore your relationship with medication is to practice gratitude. Instead of resenting the drugs and how they represent your illness, be thankful. After you have reminded yourself about the benefits of the medications, say to yourself, "I am thankful that I live in a time and place where there are scientists who develop treatments like this and doctors who know what to prescribe." In most of the world, people do not have access to the kind of care you do if you are reading this book. Practice gratitude.

Develop strategies for remembering to take your medications as prescribed, both at the right time and in the right manner. Get one (or more) of those pill containers with compartments for each day of the week. Some have four different slots for each day, so you can sort your medications by time. Choose one day of the week for filling your containers. When you fill the slots for the week, check to see if you have enough for the following week. If not, call your doctor or pharmacy and order refills. If possible, set up your prescriptions to be refilled automatically at your pharmacy. While laying out your medications, applaud yourself for being a responsible and proactive patient! "I am a good patient. I follow my treatment regimen. I am a partner in achieving my highest level of wellness."

It takes time for new ways of thinking to take hold and become part of you. You may very well practice these habits and new ways of thinking for months before you realize that you have indeed changed your attitude. In fact, once this change really sticks, you might even find yourself agitated at the thought of NOT taking your medication!

44. How can I find help to pay for my medication and other medical expenses?

The people who need medical care often face the most challenges trying to get it. Forced to stop working or reduce work hours because of illness, many chronically ill people face the double whammy of losing insurance and income at the same time. Some are simply uninsurable. Dr. Andrew P. Wilper and colleagues from the Cambridge Health Alliance/Harvard Medical School in Cambridge, Massachusetts, found that an estimated 11.5 million Americans with at least one chronic illness have no health insurance, and 22.6% had not visited a physician in the last 12 months. After the researchers adjusted for age, gender, and race or ethnicity, they found that the chronically ill uninsured patients were four to six times more likely than sick patients with insurance to have these access problems. Those who can see their doctors are likely to have a hard time paying for their prescriptions. People with chronic illness who are on Medicare can easily fall into the "doughnut hole" earlier in the yearly cycle of benefits. Those people poor enough to get Supplemental Security Income (SSI) and Medicaid are saddled with a share of cost that they usually cannot pay.

If you are one of the 11.5 million Americans who find themselves with chronic illness and no insurance, you have to fight especially hard or have someone help you fight. Check with your local health department. Services vary widely from state to state and within any given state, but this is a good starting point. Call your local county or city social services department and ask about indigent health care programs. Ask if there are any private free clinics in your area. Some local ministerial associations are able to help. Individual local houses of worship may have some limited funds as well. Ask not only about seeing a doctor but also about reduced fees for laboratory tests.

If you are one of the 11.5 million Americans who find themselves with chronic illness and no insurance, you have to fight especially hard or have someone help you fight.

Paying for medication is an enormous issue for the chronically ill. The majority of pharmaceutical companies have patient assistance programs. For many, if your family income is less than 243% of the poverty level you will qualify for some assistance. The income scale is weighted according to the income of the household and the number of people living in it. For a single person it is just over $10,000. So a person who lives alone and makes under $24,300 has a good chance of qualifying for some kind of help paying for medication. Please don't say, "I won't qualify." You won't know unless you try. The Partnership for Prescription Assistance (PPARX) is a clearing house for patient-assistance programs. Their services are free. You can call them at (888) 477-2669 or apply online at www.pparx.org/Intro.php. There are a few drug manufacturers that are not listed with PPARX. You can find the contact information for individual manufacturers at www.needymeds.org/. The Needymeds site also has a searchable database of some 3,400 free clinics and has printable coupons for medications. For a list of foundations helping with co-payments on medication, check out www.iononline.com/display.aspx?cid=CoPayAssistanceFoundations.cms. The Patient Advocate Foundation offers assistance to patients with specific issues they are facing with their insurer, employer, and/or creditor regarding insurance, job retention, and/or debt crisis matters relative to their diagnosis of life-threatening or debilitating diseases. For more information, visit www.patientadvocate.org/index.php or call (800) 532-5274.

Fight hard to find the medical care and medications that you need. When chronic illness is ignored, the results can be catastrophic. Remember, your life is valuable, and you have just as much right to live as anyone else on the planet!

PART SEVEN

Taking an Active Role in Your Own Care

How can I regain control of my health?

What is the role of positive thinking in chronic illness?

Is exercise helpful in managing chronic illness?

How can I find trustworthy information about my condition?

More . . .

45. How can I regain control of my health?

Loss of control has to be one of the most terrifying aspects of chronic illness. Your body is out of control. Emotions are frequently out of control. You are poked and prodded and invaded by medical procedures. If you want to control the disease, you have to take chemical concoctions that can cause other problems. If you don't take the drugs the disease will get more and more out of control.

There are things you can control. There are things you cannot control. The first thing to do is figure out which is which. Stop obsessing over what you can't control. All that does is make you sicker. You have control over more than you think. The doctor is not in control of your medical condition; you are. The doctor only sees you every now and then. You are with yourself and your condition 24/7. You expect your doctor to be a professional doctor. You have to be a professional patient.

46. Are there "natural" approaches that I can use to cure myself?

Most of us are willing to tolerate short-term medical interventions and courses of treatment when we know there is an end in sight. Folks with chronic diseases are on some kind of treatment regimen for the rest of their lives. Chronic illness may not be a death sentence, but it is a life sentence! Is it any wonder that patients turn away from the bearers of bad news and go off in search of magic bullets and natural cures?

Popular advertising (print, television, infomercials, and free-sample distributors in warehouse clubs) for many "natural" products on the market sell these products by generating mistrust of the medical profession. The commercials want you to believe that the medical establishment has secret information that they hide from sick people in order to make themselves rich. The theory has become so prevalent that many people actually take it to be truth. It's time for a reality check! The vast majority of doctors became doctors because they wanted to help people, not harm them by hiding cures. The supposed "natural cure" advertising implies that the drug companies and doctors merely want to get rich at the expense of suffering patients. Ask yourself, what are the sellers of "natural cures" doing? Have you ever looked into their multi-level marketing schemes? What is the evidence for their claims? Were there true scientific studies done? What methods were used? Where are the results published? Remember that hemlock and arsenic are natural too, but they can kill you (just ask Socrates!). And IF these cures worked, why are so many people still sick and suffering? Why are millions of dollars being spent on research? A sales representative for some very expensive berry juice ($25 for a quart bottle) claimed that it could cure a whole range of chronic conditions. His proof? There was something on Yahoo! A doctor recently contacted the local Lupus Foundation office claiming that he had a neuropeptide vaccination that would cure lupus. It only cost $250 a shot and might take two shots to do the trick. Of course, it wasn't approved for use in this country, and people should call his cell because he didn't maintain a physical office! I could post something on the Internet claiming that cheesecake cures cancer but that wouldn't make it true!

Herbs, vitamins, and micronutrients are often touted as cures. Think about it; as a society, we take whole food in its natural state, fragment it, refine it, then we fortify it to put back some of what we took out.

Wheat is a perfect example. We remove the fiber and bleach the wheat to make white flour. Then we add fiber to our water or yogurt to keep our bowels moving. We process the vitamins out of food and then pay lots of money to take the very same vitamins in pills. Why not eat the whole food in the first place? A word of caution: ALWAYS discuss any herb, vitamin, or supplement with your doctor BEFORE taking anything. Some of these "natural" cures can make your disease worse or have a negative interaction with your medications.

Good, whole food is the best "natural cure" you can give to your body.

What can you do to help yourself? Good, whole food is the best "natural cure" you can give to your body. Eat a healthy, balanced diet. Strive for one that is low in fat, high in fiber, and avoids too many processed foods. Get regular exercise, even if all you can do is walk or swing your arms for a few minutes. Talk to your doctor, and develop a treatment plan together. Remember, there are no magic bullets. Living your best life takes work!

47. What is a professional patient?

A professional patient is someone who takes responsibility for living the best life possible in spite of chronic illness.

A professional patient keeps good records. A professional patient follows the treatment plan. A professional patient reports accurately. And a professional patient is a good self-manager all the time. Harry, devastated by an unexpected triple coronary bypass surgery, decided to be a professional patient the day he declared, "I am going to be the best heart patient this doctor has ever had. And I am going to get better." And he did!

The questions that follow will help you become a professional patient and competent self-manager.

48. What can I do to manage fatigue?

Managing fatigue requires a three-pronged approach: identify the sources of fatigue, develop strategies for dealing with the source of fatigue, and employ energy conservation. Fatigue can be a side effect of medications, a result of irregular and interrupted sleep, lack of physical exercise, blood sugar irregularities, anemia, pain, depression, a host of other things, or a combination of factors. Put on your detective hat to figure out the sources of your fatigue. Discuss your fatigue with your doctor so that together you can rule out biological causes. If the source of your fatigue is biological, that should be addressed. If the source of your fatigue is emotional, consider counseling to deal with the underlying issues. If the source of your fatigue is a result of the side effects of medication, perhaps your doctor can prescribe an alternative. Remember, you may not be able to relieve your fatigue altogether, but with perseverance and the help of your medical team, you can identify the sources of your fatigue and develop strategies for improving the quality of your life.

Even if you have identified the sources and some solutions for your fatigue, you may still find yourself tiring easily. Three more strategies are in order here. First, examine your goals. Second, break tasks into reasonable and achievable parts. Third, be gentle with yourself and rest when you need to.

We live in a goal-oriented society. We are achievers. We ask little children what they are going to be when they grow up. It's not about now, not about being a child now, but what you are going to be later. That goal orientation remains with many of us throughout our adult lives. When we have chronic illness or disability, we may still be setting goals that are more suitable for healthy people. It's not enough for us to have the goal of living the best life possible with chronic illness. No. We have to be the one-legged marathon runner or the quadriplegic who paints the Mona Lisa with a paintbrush held in her teeth! These people are certainly inspirational, but they set a standard that is unrealistic for the vast majority of those who struggle with compromised health. When you set an unrealistic goal you are setting yourself up for failure. Each failure will erode your self-esteem until the mere thought of trying is overwhelming. Goal setting in chronic illness begins with one simple mantra, "What can I do to take care of myself right now?" Then do it!

Break tasks into smaller, manageable steps, and rest between them. Instead of cleaning an entire closet, organize just one shelf. Instead of washing and detailing your entire car, wash the inside of the windshield. Instead of cleaning the whole house at once, get up and clean during television commercials and then sit down again and rest. Write down something you want to accomplish. Break that down into steps. Break each step down into smaller steps. For example, you may want to cook dinner. What steps are involved? Decide what to cook, make sure you have the ingredients, and then cook. Right? If we break cooking dinner down we might get: decide what to cook, check ingredients, make a list of what you need, go to store, cook. And if we break it down even more? Decide what to cook, check for ingredients, get keys, get wallet, get in car, go to store, buy pasta and frozen garlic bread, get in car, come home, etc. Even little goals have many more little steps. When you break a task down to its smallest components you realize just how much you are accomplishing. When you recognize all of the small achievements that go into what seems like one simple task like cooking dinner your self-esteem will improve as you accomplish each little step.

Be gentle with yourself. Sometimes you'll make it, and sometimes you won't. That's OK. Do what you can. Rest when you need to, before you are exhausted. Don't beat yourself up for what you didn't get done; instead be thankful for what you did accomplish. Rather than keeping a "to do" list, why not try keeping an "I did it" list? If you are still having a hard time being gentle with yourself try a little game of role reversal. Pretend that you are healthy and that you care very much about someone who has your condition. What would you expect of that sick person? How would you treat him? Aren't you worthy of that kind of treatment, especially from yourself? What do YOU need to do to take care of YOURSELF right this minute?

49. What can I do to manage pain?

In order to manage pain, you have to look for the source of the pain. Most people blame their illness for their pain. The illness may be partly responsible for the pain. Other factors also contribute to pain.

Physical pain is caused by inflammation and by damage. The pain is how your body tells you that something is wrong. It is a warning designed to get your attention and protect you from further damage. Your doctor will prescribe medication to try to minimize the cause of the pain. You may also get a prescription for medication to reduce the pain. Sadly, for many people with chronic illness symptoms often go untreated, and the patient goes undiagnosed for years because of medications that only masked symptoms. Nothing was done to address the root cause.

Pain rarely occurs in isolation. Pain brings other problems. These problems in turn worsen pain. Depression can cause real physical pain. If you have chronic illness you are living with pain, fatigue, uncertainty, worry, loss of identity, and loss of control, to name just a few unpleasant feelings. Who wouldn't be depressed? Treating depression in whatever way is appropriate for you is likely to result in less pain. Muscle tension can also cause physical pain. Muscles become tense as a result of worry and anxiety. Lack of use also causes muscle pain. Fatigue brought on by the disease itself can cause pain. Pain can make sleep difficult or impossible, resulting in more pain.

Managing pain is a team effort that requires work on your part and help from your health care providers. If you don't explain your pain clearly, in language they can understand, your doctors won't be able to give you the right help. Keep a symptom journal for your pain. Include answers to these questions. When did the pain start? How often do you have pain? How long does it last? Does it vary in intensity? What makes it better? What makes it worse? On a scale of 1 to 10, with 10 being the worst, how much does your pain interfere with your ability to carry out basic activities of daily living? Describe the pain. Is it throbbing, stabbing, sharp, dull, cramping, aching, etc.?

Depression, fatigue, anxiety, fear, and muscle tension all contribute to the pain and the pain contributes to them.

You have a part in managing your pain. While the doctor can prescribe something to address the source and the symptom, you can work on the pain from your side. Depression, fatigue, anxiety, fear, and muscle tension all contribute to the pain and the pain contributes to them. Pick any one of these items and begin to work on it. Consider professional help from a counselor who specializes in pain and chronic illness. Counselors or psychologists who work with oncology practices are good choices. They work with people undergoing cancer treatments, so they understand the nature of chronic conditions.

Distraction is a valuable tool in managing not only pain, but the emotions that contribute to the pain cycle. Your mind can only concentrate on one thing at a time. If you become deeply engrossed in a movie, book, activity that you enjoy, or another person, you will find that you have forgotten your pain for that period of time. Meditation reduces stress and anxiety, leading to reduction in pain. Mild to moderate exercise releases muscle tension. Exercise also lubricates the joints, gets more oxygen into the body, removes waste, and makes your body create endorphins. All of these things reduce pain.

50. What is the role of humor in managing chronic illness?

Two nursing students were assigned to observe a disease support group as part of their studies. They came to a lupus support group. Afterward, they expressed their amazement at the amount of laughter in the group. The students had listened to the patients sharing the challenges that they faced and the many ways that lupus can affect a person's body. The patients explained that the disease had already stolen enough; they were not giving up their right to laugh. Laughter made everyone feel better.

If you have been suppressing all of the difficult emotions that travel with chronic illness, you probably haven't laughed or cried in a while. You can't suppress emotions selectively. Either you allow yourself to feel or you don't. Laughter makes you feel better. Letting yourself laugh also means you have to let yourself cry. Both are good. Difficult emotions that are kept inside make your disease worse and make your relations with others go sour. Unpleasant emotions are like radioactive waste. Each time you express them they lose half their power.

Norman Cousins, a journalist, developed ankylosing spondylitis. This is an autoimmune disease that causes arthritis or joint inflammation in the spine. It is very painful and can result in the spine fusing itself together. In his book, *Anatomy of an Illness as Perceived by the Patient*, Cousins chronicles his hospitalizations and struggles with the disease. In addition to traditional medical care, Cousins watched countless comedy movies, notably the Marx brothers. He laughed. He recovered. On the topic of laughter, Cousins said "It has always seemed to me that hearty laughter is a good way to jog internally without having to go outdoors."

Laughter reduces stress and helps manage pain. It improves mental and physical health. Humor and laughter can be used anytime and anywhere by anyone. It's free or very low cost. According to Laughter Rx, "[Laughter] is especially beneficial for those who are homebound, lack the financial resources for more expensive forms of psychotherapeutic care, do not have a strong support system, or live in areas far from pain clinics and mental health outpatient clinics." A good dose of humor can even reduce dependence on prescription painkillers and antidepressants! (A word of caution: Never stop antidepressants unless you speak with your doctor. Doing so could be very dangerous to your health.)

51. What is the role of positive thinking in chronic illness?

A hammer can be used to build or to destroy. Depending on your understanding, positive thinking can be a tool that leads toward your best life or one that beats you down. How can positive thinking be a bad thing? If positive thinking is telling yourself, "I am going to think myself out of this disease. I don't have this disease anymore," you will be disappointed, especially if you stop following your treatment plan. It certainly doesn't help when well-intentioned friends and family tell you that you just have to "think positive" and you will get well. First of all, this approach assumes that your disease is all in your head and that your head can make it go away. The second problem is New Age Guilt (NAG). You get this nagging feeling that not only are you a failure because you are sick, you are an even bigger failure because you can't positively think your way out of illness. Then you get depressed because you are a failure. Depression leads to fatigue and pain, and the downward spiral begins again. Positive thinking used the right way is an extremely valuable tool in managing chronic illness.

Norman Cousins writes, "Since the human body tends to move in the direction of its expectations—plus or minus—it is important to know that attitudes of confidence and determination are no less a part of the treatment program than medical science and technology." Positive thinking means replacing negative thoughts like, "What's the use?" with positive thoughts like, "I am going to give this a try." For just one day, or for even part of a day, make yourself aware of each negative thought and statement. Write them down. Then turn each one around and make it positive. Cousins offers this bit of wisdom, "Never deny a diagnosis, but do deny the negative verdict that may go with it."

52. What is the role of nutrition in chronic illness?

I wish I had a dollar for every newly diagnosed patient who decides that he really doesn't need or want medication; he is "going natural." That could mean vegetarian, raw foods, juicing, strange supplements, macrobiotic, or organic to name a few. Some patients will eliminate entire food groups from their diet. Still others will tell themselves that they are going to feel horrid no matter what, so they might as well eat whatever they want.

The first group of patients makes the faulty assumption that changing their diet, usually after years of neglect, will erase their chronic illness. The second group assumes that what you eat really doesn't matter. Both groups miss the mark.

A healthy and balanced diet that takes into account the special considerations for your disease is a valuable complementary, not alternative, tool for self-management. A diet that is extreme, eliminates whole food groups, or concentrates entirely on supplements can be as destructive as the diet full of junk based on the excuse that you "deserve" these treats because you are suffering.

53. What is good nutrition?

Your body is already challenged by chronic illness. Your body needs a wide variety of nutrients to maintain the best level of health possible. There is no room for empty calories. Your immune system examines every strange chemical that comes into your body trying to figure out if it is friend or foe. It makes sense to give your body good healthy food, as free of chemicals, hormones, pesticides, and preservatives as possible so that your immune system doesn't have to work overtime. One of my personal measures of whether or not I will eat something is the "rot factor." If I leave it out on the counter for days and it doesn't rot or grow "hair" I don't put it in my body. (Well, in a weak moment I might eat it!)

People with chronic illness are more likely to be sedentary. Obesity is an issue. You need all of your calories to contribute to health. Empty calories from many fats, refined sugar and flour, fast food, and prepared food coupled with lack of exercise can lead to obesity. Obesity brings its own chronic illness issues and makes existing ones worse.

A good diet is one that is varied and includes many foods. Five servings or more of fruits and vegetables a day is ideal. Limit animal fats. Have a reasonable amount of good fats in the form of olive oil, oily fish, and monosaturated fats. Trans fats and hydrogenated fats should be avoided. Focus on lean sources of protein. Eat whole grains instead of refined grains. If you plan to add supplements, always check with your doctor first! A great tool for planning your overall healthy diet can be found at www.nhlbi.nih.gov/chd/index.htm.

54. Is exercise helpful in managing chronic illness?

Exercise is extremely helpful in managing chronic illness and preventing new chronic conditions from developing. Regular physical exercise strengthens the

Exercise is extremely helpful in managing chronic illness and preventing new chronic conditions from developing.

heart muscle, brings your good and bad cholesterol into a better ratio, improves blood flow, prevents heart disease and stroke, and reduces blood pressure and body fat. Reductions in body fat help prevent and control type 2, or noninsulin-dependent, diabetes. Physical activity coupled with good, sound nutrition prevents and, over time, eliminates obesity, which is a major risk factor in many diseases. Regular exercise increases muscle strength, flexibility, and posture, helping to prevent back pain. Weight-bearing exercise improves and prevents osteoporosis, which often comes with aging or as a result of medications like prednisone. Regular exercise lubricates the joints, reduces pain, improves mood, reduces stress and anxiety, and is a valuable tool in stress management.

55. What kind of exercise should I do?

There are three basic kinds of exercise: cardiovascular, stretching, and strength. All three have a place in chronic disease self-management. Before you begin any exercise program, always talk with your doctor(s).

Exercise like walking, swimming, and biking make the heart work a little harder than normal. These are cardiovascular exercises. You will notice that your body feels warmer, and you might perspire. Your heart rate increases. A good measure of the right level of cardiovascular exercise is the talk test. You should be able to carry on a conversation while you are exercising. If you are working so hard that you can't carry on a conversation, cut back a level. But do keep in mind that this kind of exercise is moderate exertion. A leisurely stroll through the mall does not count as cardiovascular exercise.

Stretching helps maintain flexibility. Stretching reduces stress and tension. Search for stretching classes at your local gym, YMCA, community center, or senior center. Stretching helps you complete your daily tasks with less effort because you are not working against rigid muscles and tendons. Yoga is a marvelous way to do your stretching. You don't have to sit in full lotus or do a backbend. Yoga can be adapted to your level of flexibility and gradually increase it. Iyengar yoga uses props like blocks, straps, and bolsters to adapt postures and allow you to get the maximum benefit from stretching regardless of your flexibility level.

Strength training includes weights and **isometrics**. Strength training exercises increase lean muscle. When you have more lean muscle, you burn calories more efficiently. When you burn calories more efficiently you are less likely to become overweight or obese, both of which lead to complications of your disease or new chronic conditions. Some medications like prednisone can cause a decrease in bone density (**osteopenia** or **osteoporosis**). Weight-bearing exercise stresses the bones just a little bit and can prevent these conditions. Both stretching and strength training are helpful in prevention of falls that can result in injury and broken bones.

Isometrics

Exercises that involve pitting muscle against muscle or against an inanimate object (like a wall or door frame).

Osteopenia

A slight or minor thinning of the bones.

Osteoporosis

Significant thinning of the bones requiring medical treatment.

56. How can I get started with an exercise program?

When you are sick, tired, and in pain there is no desire to exercise. When depression takes over there is no desire to do anything, much less exercise. But exercise is one of the tools that can help you feel better. People fail to reach their exercise goals because they pick an exercise they don't enjoy, set unrealistic goals, don't define their goals clearly, or encounter obstacles and don't know how to overcome them. Before you attempt any exercise plan, be sure to talk with your doctor about what you intend to do.

Select physical activities that you enjoy. If you hate to be outdoors, then walking around your neighborhood is probably not the right choice for you. If you still want to walk, you can purchase videos and walk right in your living room! Make a list of all the exercises that you might do. Then go over the list and pick out the ones that you would enjoy. Remember, you want to include some cardiovascular exercise, some stretching, and some strength training. You don't have to do them all on the same day or at the same time. Think about what you need in order to do those exercises. Do you need walking shoes? Resistance bands? Light weights?

Next, set a realistic goal. If you have been a couch potato all your life, an initial goal of walking an hour a day is not realistic. If your goal is unrealistic and you fail, you are going to feel worse about yourself and probably give up altogether. Your goal is not carved in stone and can be adjusted over time. For someone who has not exercised in a long time, a 10-minute walk might be a reasonable goal. The important thing is to be realistic.

Goals must be clearly defined or you won't have any way of knowing if you achieved it or not. *I am going to get more exercise* is a vague goal. What are you going to do? How long are you going to do it? How often are you going to do it? When are you going to do it? Where are you going to do it? Here is a clear, realistic, measurable action plan:

- What are you going to do? Walk.
- How long are you going to do it? 10 minutes.
- How often are you going to do it? 3 days this week.
- When are you going to do it? After dinner.
- Where are you going to do it? On my block. If the weather is bad, I will walk in place in the living room.

It will be easy for you to know if you achieved your goal. If you find that you can't or don't achieve your goal, keep modifying it until you reach a level where you can be successful. Remember you can exceed your goal if you wish. If you walk for 10 minutes and feel like doing more, great! If not, you have reached your goal. It is far better to set a low goal and savor the success than to set a high goal and set yourself up for failure.

57. How can my mind help manage my chronic illness?

In western cultures we tend to see the mind and body as two separate entities. You already know that what is going on in your body with your chronic illness affects your mind and emotions in many ways. You might experience trouble thinking and remembering. Unpleasant emotions like anger, fear, sadness, hopelessness, and helplessness can become constant companions. These are examples of how the sickness in the body affects the mind.

The mind can also affect the body. This is not the Pollyanna notion that you can simply think away your condition. It takes work. What you think causes what you feel. What you feel affects how your body functions. If you change the way you think, then you change your feelings and change what happens in your body. For example, if you think someone or someone is threatening, you will feel stressed and defensive. It doesn't have to be a real threat. Your perception is all that matters. When you feel stressed and defensive your body releases extra adrenaline, raises blood sugar, raises blood pressure, and activates the immune system. All of this happens just because you thought. You thought you were threatened.

As with so many other things, awareness is the beginning of change. What are you telling yourself? For one day, pay attention to your thoughts and your self-talk. Write down what you are telling yourself. Take any negative or stress-producing thoughts and challenge them. For example, you could be telling yourself that this is as good as it gets and the only way to go is down. Really? How do you know? What proof do you have? Does anyone else agree with you? Challenge your thinking to see whether or not it is rational. Now write a positive statement to replace the negative and irrational one. You might say, "I am having a rough period right now, but experience has shown me that I have ups and downs with this disease. I am going to do the things I know help me feel better." You have control over what you think. You are not a victim of your thoughts unless you choose to be one. As you examine and challenge what you tell yourself, you will gradually change your thinking, which will change your feelings, which will make your body function the best it can.

You are not a victim of your thoughts unless you choose to be one.

58. What can I do to get a good night's sleep?

First, it's important to figure out what is at the root of your sleep problems. Are you in pain? Have you been sleeping a lot during the day? Are you depressed? Are you anxious and worried because of your disease? Are you getting any exercise? Do any of your medications (such as prednisone) impact your ability to sleep? Are your expectations of how long you should sleep reasonable? How much caffeine, alcohol, or tobacco do you consume each day, and what time of day do you consume it? Are you watching television or on the computer until late at night? Keep a journal of your sleep habits and what you do during each day. It doesn't have to be too terribly detailed, just enough to get a good picture of what's going on in your life. You may be able to pinpoint the reason for your sleep issues just from reviewing your writing. Do have a discussion with your doctor, but make sure you have done some homework first. Armed with this information you will be able to help the doctor come to a quicker understanding of your sleep issues and help you find a solution. Your journal may give you some clues about things that you can change and thereby improve your sleep habits.

Consider your sleep environment. Is the temperature right for you? Are your pajamas comfortable? Does your pillow support your head properly? How is your mattress? These seem like such simple solutions, but are often overlooked. It is not a good idea to sleep with the television on. The flickering light will trick your mind and body into thinking it is daytime!

Daily physical exercise helps you sleep better. If you have been avoiding exercise, you might want to give it a try. Of course, always check with your doctor first. Exercising right before bed will have the opposite effect. Your exercise should be several hours before you plan to go to sleep. Gentle stretching exercises help release tension. Some yoga postures are especially good for quieting the body and mind for sleep.

You may not realize that you are carrying tension in your body when you get into bed. Think about surrendering your body to the mattress. Personally, I use the image of being a small child cradled in my mother's lap, leaning against her chest, and feeling totally safe. Find an image that works for you.

Progressive relaxation is another wonderful tool to help you fall asleep. Once in bed, flex the muscles in different parts of the body, hold for a full minute (you can count to 60 slowly), and then release. A typical sequence would be feet and legs, then abdomen, chest, arms and hands, neck and shoulders, and finally the face.

Any adult who has cared for young children learns quickly that a regular bedtime routine helps the little ones settle down and fall asleep. It really isn't that much different with us. The first thing to do is to keep a consistent schedule of bedtime and getting up. Your body actually "learns" this schedule. A couple of hours before your intended sleep time, start to wind down. This is not a time to exercise, solve major problems, or get overstimulated by violence or horror on the television (or the news, for that matter!) This is a time to prepare yourself for deep, restorative sleep. Take a warm bath. Have a snack. Quiet your mind. Before you begin your bedtime ritual, you might want to jot down anything you want to remember for the next day. Once you have a written reminder, you won't have to listen to the mental reminders that keep you awake. Play a recording of ambient, relaxing music as you go to sleep. Soon the evening bedtime ritual will trigger sleep. It almost goes without saying that if you sleep until noon, you will not be ready to sleep at 9:00 p.m. Consistent waking times are important if you want to have a consistent sleeping time.

If you try all of these techniques and still can't sleep, have an honest discussion with your doctor. There are prescription sleep aids available that carry a very limited chance of causing dependency.

Frances R.'s comment:

It's so confusing. I was newly diagnosed. The doctor didn't really explain what I could expect. So there I was, sitting in his waiting room. I struck up a conversation with another patient. When she found out what I had, she went on to describe, in great detail, how a friend of hers had the same disease and how she died a slow, lingering death as one by one her organs failed. One of my co-workers told me I might as well quit working now because my disease would make me too tired. A neighbor told me about somebody else who cured themselves just by changing their diet. They can't all be telling the truth. I just don't know what to believe.

59. How can I find trustworthy information about my condition?

When you are diagnosed with chronic illness, it seems like everyone knows someone who knows someone who has your condition. Nearly everyone around becomes an instant medical expert. They will tell you stories about people who died miserable deaths from your condition. They will tell you stories about people who have cured themselves by (pick one or add your own) going organic, eating only raw foods, taking supplements, buying and using any of the many snake oil products out there that are little more than glorified juice in expensive bottles, exercising, resting, getting more sun, getting less sun, finding a guru or a faith healer, magnets, and on and on. And then, of course, there is the Internet! You can find "cures" for virtually any disease on the Internet. The problem is they don't work. Let's be honest. No one wants to be on medication for life. No one wants to hear that their disease is here for the duration. No one wants constant medical interventions. It's easy to grasp at straws when you hear about a "miracle cure." The prevalent conspiracy theory that doctors don't want you to know simple things that will cure you fuels the desire to try "miracle cures." The only thing that gets cured is the emptiness of the pockets of the people who sell most of this stuff.

When confronted with cures that seem too good to be true, remember, they probably are. Consider the source of the information. If you are hearing about this third-hand from the checkout clerk in the grocery store whose second cousin's step-sister twice-removed cured shingles by eating marigolds, you might want to think twice. Infomercials are designed to sell you things, not necessarily give you good, solid information. Advertisements on the Internet are just that—advertisements designed to get you to buy products. So, if you can't trust your friends and family, and you can't trust the television or radio, and you can't trust the Internet, where CAN you get reliable information?

The first place to go for information is your doctor. Although the doctor can't spend hours explaining every nuance of your disease, the doctor can give you an overview, answer you most pressing questions, and point you in the direction of reliable information. Always respect the doctor's time, but also be a persistent patient. One patient on the occasion of her visit to the doctor shortly after her release from the hospital had about three questions that were very significant. Will this kill me? Is it progressive? Is my functional life over? The doctor left the room before answering the second question. The patient, a pretty tenacious lady, found him in the hallway, put her hand in his lab coat pocket to stop him from escaping and said, "Wait a minute. I'm not finished with you!" Although we certainly can't recommend that kind of behavior, the patient did get her questions answered. You can bring your most pressing questions to your appointment. You can even fax them to the doctor a few days in advance of your appointment. If the doctor seems rushed and in a hurry to get to other patients, ask for an appointment where you can have

15 minutes of undivided time to ask your questions and have them answered.

A reliable source of information is the disease foundation that is specific to what you have. You can call and ask that information be sent to you. Virtually every disease foundation has a presence on the Internet. They almost always end with dot org (.org). The United States government's National Institutes of Health is an umbrella for many specialized disease departments. Web sites that end in dot gov (.gov) are reliable. Institutions of higher learning that also conduct medical research and education will have sites ending in dot edu (.edu). Again, these sites can be trusted. If you have questions about what you have read, ask your doctor. Open and trusting communication between doctor and patient is one of the most effective tools for educating yourself and managing your chronic illness. You will find a list of resources in the appendix.

Open and trusting communication between doctor and patient is one of the most effective tools for educating yourself and managing your chronic illness.

PART EIGHT

Stress

What is the role of stress in chronic illness?

How can I manage stress that cannot be avoided?

How can meditation be used to reduce stress and manage chronic illness?

More . . .

60. What is the role of stress in chronic illness?

Life is stressful. Life with chronic illness is even more stressful. Stress makes your heart rate increase and your blood pressure go up so that the brain gets more blood to improve decision making. Stress makes your blood sugar rise to create more fuel for energy. Blood is diverted from digestion to the arms and legs in preparation for fight or flight. Blood clots more easily in case you get cut or bleed internally. Stress also affects the immune system. Chronic stress can cause any and every system in the body to break down. These bodily reactions happen whether the stress is good or bad. Herbert Benson, MD, founding president of the Mind Body Medical Institute at Beth Israel Deaconess Medical Center in Boston, and author of *The Relaxation Response*, puts it this way, "Stress comes from any situation or circumstance that requires behavioral adjustment. Any change, either good or bad, is stressful, and whether it's a positive or negative change, the physiology is the same." Stress can cause disease. Stress can make a disease worse. Stress can add diseases and disorders to what you already have.

61. How can I reduce stress in my life?

The first step to any change is awareness. Stress is very subjective. For one person, a fast and steep roller coaster is a stress reliever and a pleasure. For another person it is one of the most stressful things on the planet. Become aware of the things that cause stress for you. Write down your stressors over the course of 1 to 2 weeks. Take some quiet time and think about each stressor. What caused the stress? Was it something another person did or said? Was it an event beyond your control? Was it preventable? Did you play a part in creating your own stress? Was the stress a result of your thinking? What other things trigger stress for you?

Review your list again. This time put each stressor into one of two categories: things you can change and things you can't change. Select one of the more common stressors on your list that fall into the category of changeable. Make a list of all the things you could do to change that stressor. Each time you are faced with that stressor or possibility of it, do something from your list to change it.

There are stressors that you can't control. However, you can control your reaction to these stressors. Imagine that you are stuck in a long line at the grocery store. You can't control the length of the line or the speed of the cashiers. If you choose to get agitated, mumble angrily about the wait, and seethe inside, you have chosen a reaction that is stress-full. If you choose to use the time to practice mindful breathing, people watch, or make a mental list of the things for which you are thankful, you have chosen a stress-less reaction. Go back to your list and look at the stressors that you marked as beyond your control. How can you choose a different reaction? Review these notes often so the new choices will become part of you.

Worrying about the future and dwelling in the past both cause stress. Planning for the future and worrying about the future are not the same thing. Worrying about the future will not change it for the better but the stress it creates will probably make you sicker! Reliving the past can be stressful too. If you relive something that you did that you believe to be wrong, you will agonize over it. Agonizing over past mistakes and hurts won't change what happened. If you did something to hurt someone, apologize, and let it go. If someone hurt you, forgive them, and let it go. If you relive times when you believe other people wronged you, you are only creating stress by nurturing anger and resentment. The only person you are hurting then is yourself. Again, awareness is the beginning of change. Notice how often you find your thoughts dwelling in the future or the past. When that happens, gently bring yourself back to the present moment.

In this moment, right this very second, is anything happening to stress you? If nothing stressful is happening to you at this moment, then let go of stressful thoughts. Yesterday is a cancelled check. Tomorrow is a promissory note. Today is cash in hand. Spend it wisely. You will have less stress and better health!

62. How can I manage stress that cannot be avoided?

If you are alive, you have stress. Some stresses can be reduced or eliminated. Others are unavoidable. I have never met a person who was jubilant at the prospect of an invasive medical procedure. When you experience stress, a series of chemical and hormonal changes take place in your body. Your body still responds to stress in primitive ways. Although we are rarely threatened by wild beasts hoping to have us for lunch, our bodies still react as if that was the case. This is the fight-or-flight response. Our bodies prepare us for battle with the stressful threat or to run for our lives. If we don't fight physically and we don't run, the stress chemicals remain in our bodies wreaking havoc. Movement removes these chemicals.

Just as stress is subjective, so are the ways to manage stress. Volumes have been written on the subject. Exercise releases stress and causes your body to create endorphins, which reduce pain and elevate mood. Ancient practices like yoga, Tai Chi, and Qigong calm body and mind and release stress. If you aren't able to go to a gym or yoga studio, excellent videos and DVDs are available. Good nutrition helps in the management of stress. Meditation, affirmations, visualization, and guided imagery are excellent tools in the management of stress. Massage is wonderful for managing stress. If you can't afford a massage, look for a massage education program at your community college or vocational school. You can get a student massage for as little as $20! *The Relaxation Response* by Herbert Benson, MD and *Full Catastrophe Living: Using the Wisdom of Your Body and Mind to Face Stress, Pain and Illness* by Jon Kabat-Zinn offer very clear and easy-to-follow directions for achieving a deep state of calm and relaxation. The important thing is to find the stress management techniques that work for you!

63. How can meditation be used to reduce stress and manage chronic illness?

Our minds are always thinking. Stop reading right now, and try not to think! Hard, isn't it? Where did your thoughts lead you? We relive the past. We worry about the future. Our thoughts frequently create stress. Stress doesn't have to be a real threat. If we perceive something as stressful, then it is. In the face of stress, our sympathetic nervous system kicks into high gear. In the face of stress, a cascade of chemical reactions occurs throughout the body. Living in a constant state of stress, much of which is caused by your thinking, causes chronic illnesses and makes the illnesses that you have worse.

Meditation calms the mind. Calming the mind calms the body. Calming the body leads to better health.

According to Benson, the more often the stress response is activated, the more likely you are to develop chronic high blood pressure over time. High blood pressure leads to heart attacks and strokes. One significant benefit of meditation is the lowering of blood pressure.

When you have a chronic illness, you are likely to spend a lot of time thinking about your health. You think about what you were once able to do. You feel anger, sadness, frustration, and loss because you can no longer do those things. You think about what the future may have in store for you. You worry about finances and losing your independence and becoming an invalid or losing your mind. If you happen to be thinking about what is happening right now, you are probably listing your pain and other symptoms. All of this thinking causes stress. Every minute you spend thinking about these things is a minute of your life that you have wasted!

The calm that you experience during meditation remains with you after the practice.

Meditation teaches you to quiet the thoughts and to focus on being truly present in this minute. Meditation raises awareness of body and mind. The calm that you experience during meditation remains with you after the practice. The ability to focus on one thing at a time carries over into your daily life, further reducing stress and thereby improving your overall health.

64. How can I learn to meditate?

Many people think that meditation is very mysterious or that you have to go study with Zen masters or Buddhist monks to learn it. That is not true. Although meditation is part of many spiritual practices, you can learn it apart from a specific religious path and still experience many of the health benefits. Benson studied the effects of stress and of meditation in the laboratories of Harvard Medical School and Boston's Beth Israel Hospital. His book, *The Relaxation Response*, first published in 1975, is a very useful guide to basic meditation. "Once learned, the relaxation response takes only 10 to 20 minutes twice a day and, as millions have already discovered, can relieve the restlessness and tension that stand between you and a richer, fuller, healthier life."

Meditation requires no special equipment. You can do it anywhere. One of the simplest ways is known as following the breath. Find a quiet place. Wear loose, comfortable clothing. You can sit or lie down, just make sure you are comfortable. If you are sitting in a chair, make sure your feet are both flat on the floor. Close your eyes. Breathe in and out slowly through the nose (unless, of course, your nose is stuffed.) Notice the sensation of the air moving into your body. Notice the sensation of the air leaving your body. Continue to observe your own breathing and the sensations in your body. Your mind will probably wander off and start thinking. That's OK. Observe that your mind has done this and then gently bring it back to following the breath.

You can count while breathing. Mentally count to four as you breathe in and again as you breathe out. As before, if your mind goes off on its own, notice that, and bring the mind gently back to the breath. Some people find it helpful to use prayer with the breath. Breathe in, noticing the feelings of breathing in, then as you exhale think one line of a prayer that you know.

There are numerous books and CDs available that can guide you through a meditation session. The Center for Mindfulness at the University of Massachusetts has excellent CDs for mindfulness-based stress reduction (see Appendix for more information). You might want to consider checking some out from your local library first so that you can preview them and later purchase those that work for you.

PART NINE

Clinical Trials

What are clinical trials?

What are the risks and benefits of clinical trials?

How can I find clinical trials?

More . . .

65. What are clinical trials?

The journey for new medications is a long one. The journey starts with an idea and ends up in your local pharmacy. New medications are tested in the laboratory and then on animals before moving on to clinical trials involving humans. Clinical trials may be sponsored by individuals, physicians, medical institutions, or voluntary groups such as disease foundations, drug companies, and government agencies.

People have different reasons for wanting to participate in clinical trials. "Participants in clinical trials can play a more active role in their own health care, gain access to new research treatments before they are widely available, and help others by contributing to medical research," according to ClinicalTrials.gov. Not everyone can participate in a clinical trial. There are very specific criteria for who can be included and who will be excluded. The researchers have to put these restrictions in place so that they can have the best data in determining the effectiveness of a new treatment.

There are different kinds of clinical trials. Treatment trials test various kinds of experimental treatments. Prevention trials examine ways to prevent a disease for people who have never had it, or stop a disease from returning. Diagnostic trials seek to find better ways to diagnose particular diseases, while screening trials test the best way to detect certain diseases or health conditions. And finally, quality-of-life trials are designed to look for ways to improve the quality of life for people with chronic diseases.

According to ClinicalTrials.gov, clinical trials have different phases, each involving more participants.

- Phase I trials: Researchers test an experimental drug or treatment in a small group of people (20 to 80) for the first time to evaluate its safety, determine a safe dosage range, and identify side effects.
- Phase II trials: The experimental study drug or treatment is given to a larger group of people (100 to 300) to see if it is effective and to further evaluate its safety.
- Phase III trials: The experimental study drug or treatment is given to large groups of people (1000 to 3000) to confirm its effectiveness, monitor side effects, compare it to commonly used treatments, and collect information that will allow the experimental drug or treatment to be used safely.
- Phase IV trials: Post-marketing studies delineate additional information including the drug's risks, benefits, and optimal use.

66. What are the risks and benefits of clinical trials?

Clinical trials have benefits. You may get access to new treatments before they are available to the general public. You get to play a very active role in your own health care. You can get expert medical care during the trial. And you have the satisfaction of knowing that you are contributing to medical research that may end up helping millions of people.

Clinical trials also have risks. In some kinds of trials you may receive a placebo and not get the study medication at all. This is necessary so that the researchers can truly measure the efficacy of the treatment. If you get the placebo, your disease could worsen. The treatment medications might have serious or life-threatening side effects. Or you may find that following the trial protocol is more involved and time-consuming than you are willing to endure. If you are accepted for a clinical trial, you always have the option of leaving the trial.

67. How can I find clinical trials?

The best way to find clinical trials is to go to www. ClinicalTrials.gov. The database of trials is searchable by condition, location, drug intervention, and sponsor. The National Institutes of Health suggest the following for people considering clinical trials:

People should know as much as possible about the clinical trial and feel comfortable asking the members of the health care team questions about it, the care expected while in a trial, and the cost of the trial. The following questions might be helpful for the participant to discuss with the health care team. Some of the answers to these questions are found in the informed consent document.

- What is the purpose of the study?
- Who is going to be in the study?
- Why do researchers believe the experimental treatment being tested may be effective? Has it been tested before?
- What kinds of tests and experimental treatments are involved?
- How do the possible risks, side effects, and benefits in the study compare with my current treatment?
- How might this trial affect my daily life?
- How long will the trial last?
- Will hospitalization be required?
- Who will pay for the experimental treatment?
- Will I be reimbursed for other expenses?
- What type of long-term follow-up care is part of this study?
- How will I know that the experimental treatment is working? Will results of the trials be provided to me?
- Who will be in charge of my care?

PART TEN

Special Considerations for Common Chronic Illnesses

What is autoimmunity?

How do I know if alcohol or other substances have become a chronic illness for me?

What is COPD?

What can I do to about high blood pressure?

More . . .

Dennis D.'s comment:

I get so tired of people telling me that I don't look sick! What does sick look like anyway? I do my best to be presentable, just like anyone else. I take a shower, comb my hair, and wear clean clothes. Just because my disease doesn't show on the outside doesn't mean it's not doing bad things on the inside. And just because I don't look sick, doesn't mean I don't feel sick. I used to work in our family business. I was a real go-getter, putting in long days. After I got sick, I was lucky to put in 3 hours a day. My brother, who happens to be very smart and well-educated, got mad because I wasn't pulling my weight anymore. He told me I didn't look sick. And I told him that he didn't look stupid either!

68. What is invisible chronic illness?

Invisible chronic illnesses (ICI) present a special set of challenges. If you have an ICI not only do you have to live with the illness, but also with the fact that your illness is invisible. You don't look sick! Other people cannot see symptoms like pain, confusion, fatigue, or subtle changes in memory and cognition. These symptoms are difficult for medical professionals to measure if the symptoms can be measured at all. People, including doctors, doubt that the patient is truly sick. They may attribute the problems to stress, overwork, or depression. In short, invisible can easily be dismissed as "being all in your head." Indeed, people with ICI doubt themselves, especially if their illness, like many chronic illnesses, has periods of activity and relative calm.

The absence of visible and measurable symptoms results in patients being sick for years before they are taken seriously enough to get a diagnosis.

The absence of visible and measurable symptoms results in patients being sick for years before they are taken seriously enough to get a diagnosis. ICI is very difficult to diagnose. Clinicians are forced to rely on subjective descriptions of the symptoms provided by the patient. And the truth is that some of these symptoms occur as part of mental illness. A doctor may make an attempt, but without any measurable clinical evidence, no diagnosis is made. In the meantime, the disease continues to progress, often causing permanent damage.

In *Sick and Tired of Feeling Sick and Tired: Living with Invisible Chronic Illness,* Donoghue and Siegel list some of the more baffling and prevalent invisible chronic illnesses: arthritis, which includes some 100 conditions, Charcot-Marie-Tooth disease (**neuropathy** and muscular dystrophy), chronic fatigue immune dysfunction syndrome, endometriosis, fibromyalgia, human immunodeficiency virus (HIV), inflammatory bowel disease, irritable bowel syndrome, systemic lupus erythematosus, Lyme disease, migraine, multiple sclerosis, post-polio syndrome, premenstrual syndrome, and thyroid illnesses. Many of the autoimmune diseases can also be included in this list.

Neuropathy
Nerve pain.

Perhaps one of the most difficult challenges of ICI is doubt and suspicion. Doctors doubt the validity of your symptoms. Family, friends, and co-workers cannot see any tangible evidence of the illness and suspect the patient of faking sickness to get out of work, to get out of commitments, or because the patient is simply a hypochondriac. In the face of all this doubt and suspicion, the patient likewise begins to doubt the reality of the illness, especially in illnesses that have a remitting/flaring nature. The doubt coming at you from both outside of you and within you leads to increased stress and insecurity, making whatever you have even worse.

69. What is autoimmunity?

Autoimmunity is a condition in which the immune system is unable to tell the difference between healthy parts of the self and invaders such as bacteria, viruses, and parasites. According to Douglas Kerr in a Foreword to *The Autoimmune Epidemic* by Donna Jackson Nakazawa:

The numbers are staggering: 1 in 12 Americans—and 1 in 9 women—will develop an autoimmune disorder. And since it is clear that not every patient with an autoimmune disease is correctly diagnosed, the prevalence is certainly higher than that. The American Heart Association estimates that by comparison, only 1 in 20 Americans will have coronary heart disease. Similarly, according to the National Center for Health Statistics, 1 in 14 American adults will have cancer at some time in their life. This means that an American is more likely to get an autoimmune disease than either cancer or heart disease.

Some autoimmune diseases are rather specialized, attacking just one part of the healthy self. Others, like systemic lupus erythematosus, aren't so picky. They are equal-opportunity destroyers, going after any part of the body. Autoimmune diseases can be hard to diagnose not only because of the subjective nature of the symptoms but also because they like to travel with other autoimmune conditions. If you have one autoimmune disease, you probably have others. This has led some scientists to consider the notion that there is one disease—autoimmunity—that takes on many different manifestations.

The American Autoimmune Related Diseases Association lists over 100 autoimmune and related disorders. Many people are surprised when they find out just how many diseases are autoimmune. Here are a few: alopecia, celiac disease–sprue, Crohn's disease, type 1 diabetes, Graves' disease and Hashimoto's thyroiditis, juvenile arthritis, multiple sclerosis, psoriasis and psoriatic arthritis, rheumatoid arthritis, and Sjögren's syndrome. Many other diseases are suspected of having their basis in autoimmunity.

70. How are autoimmune diseases managed?

At this time, there are no cures for autoimmune diseases. There are treatment goals, however. **Immunosuppressive drugs** are used to calm and weaken the immune system and prevent long-term damage. Cancer chemotherapies whose side effect is to weaken the immune system are sometimes used to treat autoimmune diseases. Newer drugs for the treatment of autoimmunity include biologics. Biologics are genetically engineered proteins from human genes and are designed to target very specific parts of the immune system. These same drugs may address the cause of the symptoms. For symptoms like pain and neuropathy, other medications may be included to minimize the symptoms further. Earlier immunosuppressive drugs could be likened to tossing a hand grenade into the body to disrupt the autoimmune activity. Newer drugs are more specific and can target the immune system problems in more particular ways. Much research still needs to be done. Nakazawa addresses the need for more funding for autoimmune research: "Though the NIH [National Institutes of Health] has expanded funding for autoimmunity significantly over the last several years, the 2003 expenditure of $591.2 million is still only a fraction of the money spent for heart disease and cancer. The NIH budget for cancer is over 5 billion dollars ... for cardiovascular disease [the budget] is over 2 billion dollars."

Immunosuppressive drugs

Drugs designed to treat autoimmunity by weakening a person's immune system.

Regular medical monitoring is essential in managing autoimmune disease. The autoimmune activity can increase, causing permanent damage of which the patient may be unaware. Medications are adjusted to reflect changes in the level of disease activity.

The patient's role in managing autoimmunity is crucial. Since stress stimulates the immune system, the patient must learn to reduce stress whenever possible and manage the stress that cannot be reduced (see Question 62). In addition to managing stress, a healthy diet is essential. One of the results of autoimmune disease is inflammation, which includes inflammation of the blood vessels. High blood pressure and atherosclerosis (hardening of the arteries) can result. Steroids are commonly used as a first line of defense in the presence of inflammatory autoimmune disease. Steroids cause weight gain, exacerbating the risk of heart attack, stroke, and high blood pressure. A healthy eating plan and maintaining optimal weight help reduce these risks. Minimizing artificial additives is wise. Each time the immune system encounters a substance that is a human-made chemical, it has to figure out if this chemical is safe or hurtful. If you give your immune system a lot of these chemicals, it will be stressed trying to figure out what to do.

Each time the immune system encounters a substance that is a human-made chemical, it has to figure out if this chemical is safe or hurtful.

71. What is my diabetes risk?

Type 1 diabetes often occurs at an early age and is unpredictable. This kind of diabetes is autoimmune. The pancreas is attacked and stops making insulin.

Type 2 diabetes may develop as a result of a combination of genetics and lifestyle.

Known risk factors that may increase your risk for type 2 diabetes:

- Age greater than 45 years
- Excess body weight (especially around the waist)
- Family history of diabetes
- Diabetes during a past pregnancy
- Giving birth to a baby weighing more than 9 pounds
- Low levels of **HDL**, the "good" cholesterol in the blood-stream
- High levels of triglycerides, a type of fat in the blood-stream
- High blood pressure (greater than or equal to 140/90 mmHg)
- Pre-diabetes
- Low activity level
- Poor diet

HDL

High-density lipoprotein, or "good" cholesterol.

72. Is there an online tool to check for diabetes?

Diabetes PHD (Personal Health Divisions), offered by the American Diabetes Association, is an interactive risk-assessment tool on its Web site. To complete a Diabetes PHD analysis, visit www.diabetes.org/diabetesphd. You will be asked to enter as much as you can about your health history and medications. Once completed, Diabetes PHD measures your future risk for developing diabetes, heart attack, stroke, kidney failure, and foot and eye complications.

You can change certain variables in your profile, such as losing weight or quitting smoking, to see how making positive changes will improve your future health.

73. How can exercise help with my diabetes?

- Help you feel better physically and mentally
- Improve your strength, flexibility, and endurance
- Help your insulin work better
- Lower your blood glucose, blood pressure, and cholesterol
- Reduce your risk for heart disease and stroke
- Strengthen your heart, muscles, and bones
- Improve your blood circulation and keep your joints flexible
- Exercise can lower your blood glucose for many hours and is beneficial for your heart, muscles, mood, weight, and confidence.

If you are considering an exercise program, consult your doctor first to determine a plan that will work for you.

74. What is osteoporosis?

Even though they may not look like it, our bones are living, growing structures. Old bone cells die and new ones replace them for as long as we live. Over time, bone cells may die faster than they are replaced. The result is osteoporosis, or thinning of the bones.

Osteoporosis is the leading cause of hip and spinal fractures. Fractures of the hip can cause permanent disability, increased hospitalization, and can lead to other serious complications. Women are affected by osteoporosis more than men because they tend to be smaller in structure and therefore have less bone mass. Menopause decreases estrogen production in women and as a result causes bone loss to occur more quickly. Some people will be able to manage their osteoporosis with diet and exercise, and others may require treatment with prescription medication. Your doctor will use your complete medical history to give you treatment options.

75. What are risk factors for osteoporosis?

- Family history of osteoporosis
- Smoking (smoking is linked to bone loss)
- Weighing less than 127 pounds (the lighter you are, the less demand you put on bones and the weaker they become)
- Early menopause before age 45 and low estrogen levels for women
- Low testosterone in men
- Excessive alcohol use (drinking too much alcohol can cause nutritional deficiencies)
- Long-term use of steroids

76. What can I do to manage osteoporosis?

Testing

Early testing is important. Although we have good treatments for osteoporosis, there is no cure. You can have your bone mineral density tested in a non-invasive manner.

Eat Healthy

The body needs calcium to build bone. Make sure your diet is rich in calcium by eating green vegetables, like broccoli and spinach. Dairy products are a great source of calcium. Your body needs vitamin D in order for your bones to absorb calcium. Most fortified dairy products contain vitamin D, but other sources include sunlight exposure, egg yolks, saltwater fish, and liver. If you have trouble getting enough calcium and vitamin D, calcium and vitamin D supplements might be helpful.

Stay Active

Weight-bearing exercise and resistance training can help build and maintain strong bones. Aerobic exercise can also keep bones healthy. Exercise signals your body to strengthen bone. Jogging, walking, dancing, and stair climbing are all good ways to stay active. Adding even a little resistance to your aerobic exercise will help build stronger bones. Check with your doctor before beginning any exercise plan.

77. How do I know if alcohol or other substances have become a chronic illness for me?

You can use several tools to detect a loss of control with alcohol use. The CAGE questionnaire is one such example. The questionnaire asks the following questions:

- C: Have you ever felt you needed to **Cut** down on your drinking?
- A: Have people **Annoyed** you by criticizing your drinking?
- G: Have you ever felt **Guilty** about drinking?
- E: Have you ever felt you needed a drink first thing in the morning (**Eye-opener**) to steady your nerves or to get rid of a hangover?

Two "yes" responses indicate that your behavior should be investigated further.

If you suspect that you have a problem, then you probably do.

78. What can I do to manage a substance abuse problem?

Alcohol, some prescription medications, and the so-called "recreational drugs" can be addictive. If you suspect that you have a problem, then you probably do.

No approach to ending addiction will work unless the person wants it to work. If you are trying to quit because your spouse, friends, boss, parents, or children want you to, you are not likely to succeed. When the decision is yours, when you are doing this because you want it for yourself, you have a high chance of success.

The popular myth that no one gets clean and sober until they hit bottom is just that, a myth. People change when it is too painful to stay where they are. Some people recognize that pain sooner than others. Some people try to numb the pain instead. After the decision is made to change, what next?

Twelve-step programs exist for nearly every addiction. They work. Even if someone goes to a rehabilitation facility, they will be working a twelve-step-program. In some cases, doctors may be part of the solution, providing medications that ease the difficulty that some people experience when they withdraw from the substance. The first step is an admission that your life is out of control because of (fill in the blank). From there, you work through the other steps, often with the help of a sponsor who has been through the program. The last step is helping others who are experiencing the same problem. The steps work because people learn from one another. Twelve-step groups are anonymous. No one is going to tell your doctor or family or anyone else.

79. What is COPD?

COPD stands for chronic obstructive pulmonary disease. It is a disease that starts slowly and gets worse over time. COPD makes it difficult for people to breathe. Tobacco smoke is the leading cause of COPD, but it can also be caused by pollutants, chemical fumes, or dust. Emphysema results from damage to the small air sacs in the lungs. Chronic obstructive bronchitis is an inflammation of the airways. Both are part of COPD, and both make breathing difficult and inefficient. According to the National Heart, Lung, and Blood Institute, "COPD is a major cause of disability, and it's the fourth leading cause of death in the United States. More than 12 million people are currently diagnosed with COPD. An additional 12 million likely have the disease and don't even know it."

Symptoms of COPD begin long before the disease is problematic enough to prompt someone to get medical attention. A cough that is ongoing and produces a lot of mucous, shortness of breath especially after activity, and wheezing and tightness in the chest are all symptoms of COPD. Since other diseases can cause the same symptoms, it's a good idea to talk to your doctor about COPD.

80. What can I do to manage COPD?

The goals of treatment are to relieve your symptoms, slow the progress of the disease, improve your exercise tolerance, prevent and treat complications, and improve your overall health. Your doctor may prescribe medications and vaccinations. Medications open your airways. Inhaled steroids can be helpful. Vaccinations prevent complications from things like flu and pneumonia. Pulmonary (lung) rehabilitation engages a team of health professionals. Oxygen therapy can be given periodically or constantly to people with COPD. In some cases, you might need surgery or other interventions to manage complications brought on by COPD.

Although COPD requires medical management, you have a very important role. First and foremost, if you still smoke, stop! Ninety percent of all deaths from COPD can be attributed to smoking! Quitting smoking will slow the progress of the disease. Try to avoid lung irritants. If pollution is high, stay indoors with the windows closed. Follow the treatment plan the doctor has prescribed for you. Don't hesitate to call the doctor or go to the hospital if symptoms worsen. Remember, COPD is the fourth leading cause of death in the United States. Manage the disease and its symptoms. Your doctor is your best ally in managing COPD, but you are the one who has to follow through.

81. How can I stop smoking?

COPD isn't the only chronic disease that is caused by smoking. Cigarette smoke harms every organ in the body. Scientists have proven that cigarette smoke is directly linked to leukemia, cataracts, pneumonia, and about one-third of cancer deaths. It has also been well documented that smoking substantially increases the risk of heart disease, including stroke, heart attack, vascular disease, and aneurysm. It is estimated that smoking accounts for approximately 21% of deaths from coronary heart disease each year. Smoking raises "bad" cholesterol and makes blood platelets more likely to stick together, resulting in dangerous clots. Cigarette smoking kills an estimated 440,000 U.S. citizens each year—more than alcohol, cocaine, heroin, homicide, suicide, car accidents, fire, and AIDS combined. Since 1964, more than 12 million Americans have died prematurely from smoking, and another 25 million U.S. smokers alive today will most likely die of a smoking-related illness, according to the National Institute on Drug Abuse.

Even though the clear dangers of smoking are widely known, people continue to smoke. Why? Simply put, they are addicted to nicotine, and addictions are not logical. No one wakes up in the morning and thinks, "I am so glad I am addicted to nicotine," or "Today I think it would be nice to get addicted to something." Once addicted, the first step to breaking that addiction is to truly want to be free of the addictive substance. Once you have made that decision, there are a number of options.

Some people are able to quit smoking without much assistance. Others need different forms of help. Nicotine replacement therapies deliver controlled amounts of nicotine, the addictive substance in cigarette smoke, to help minimize cravings. These therapies are available over the counter in the form of patches, gum, and lozenges. Your doctor can also prescribe some medications that can help you quit. A pill or a patch alone won't make you smoke-free. The other essential part of quitting is the use of behavioral interventions. Traditionally, behavioral approaches were developed and delivered through formal settings, such as smoking-cessation clinics and community and public health settings. Over the past decade, however, researchers have been adapting these approaches for mail, telephone, and Internet formats, which can be more acceptable and accessible to smokers who are trying to quit. In 2004, the U.S. Department of Health and Human Services (HHS) established a national toll-free number, (800) QUIT-NOW [(800) 784-8669)], to serve as a single access point for smokers seeking information and assistance in quitting. Callers are routed to their state's smoking cessation quitline or, in states that have not established quitlines, to a quitline maintained by the National Cancer Institute. In addition, a new HHS Web site (www.smokefree.gov) offers online advice and downloadable information to make cessation easier.

Quitting smoking can be difficult. While people can be helped during the time an intervention is delivered, most intervention programs are short term (1 to 3 months). Within 6 months, 75% to 80% of people who try to quit smoking relapse. National Institute for Drug Addiction research has now shown that extending treatment beyond the typical duration of a smoking cessation program can produce quit rates as high as 50% at 1 year.

You have the highest chance for success if you tailor your cessation program to your unique needs. If you fail, be gentle with yourself and begin again. The keys are the desire to quit, multiple supports, and persistence. Keep at it, and you will succeed. You will be rewarded with better health as the negative health effects of smoking begin to reverse themselves in as little as 24 hours after stopping. Talk to your doctor about quitting. Some people feel ashamed to discuss addiction with their health care providers. Your doctors want you to have the best life possible. They can help you, but only if you are honest.

Your doctors want you to have the best life possible.

82. What is my cardiovascular risk?

The American Heart Association groups risk factors into two categories: those that cannot be changed and those that can. As you age, your risk of coronary heart disease increases. Over 83% of people who die of coronary heart disease are 65 or older. In general, men have a greater risk of heart attack but women also have heart attacks. Heredity and race also factor into the risk level. African Americans, Mexican Americans, Native Americans, native Hawaiians, and some Asian Americans have increased risk as well. This is partly due to higher rates of diabetes.

Other risk factors can be reduced through lifestyle changes and/or medication. People who smoke are two to four times more likely to develop coronary heart disease than non-smokers. People who smoke cigars or pipes have a greater risk than the general population but somewhat less than cigarette smokers. Secondhand smoke also increases the chance of heart attacks!

High blood cholesterol and high blood pressure often occur together and increase the risk of coronary heart disease. When they exist with other risk factors like smoking, obesity, and diabetes, the risk of heart attack or stroke increases several times.

Other risk factors include physical inactivity, being overweight or obese, and diabetes mellitus. Stress and alcohol contribute to coronary heart disease as well. If you have these risk factors, you can modify your lifestyle and reduce your risk. If you don't have these risk factors, a healthy lifestyle can help prevent them. The American Heart Association has online tools for assessing your personal risk for heart attack and stroke along with a variety of quizzes and fact sheets on factors that influence heart health (www.ameicanheart.org).

83. What can I do to manage cholesterol?

LDL

Low-density lipoprotein, or "bad" cholesterol.

There are two types of cholesterol: "good" (HDL) and "bad" (**LDL**). Too much of the bad or not enough of the good puts you at risk for coronary heart disease, stroke, or heart attack. Your liver and other cells make about 75% of the cholesterol circulating in your body, while the food you eat contributes about 25%. Your body uses cholesterol to produce cell membranes and some hormones and is involved in other needed bodily functions. But too much puts you at risk for cardiovascular disease. The cholesterol can build up inside the walls of your blood vessels, resulting in high blood pressure. Arteries can become so clogged that they are completely blocked.

Because of genetics, some people's bodies make too much cholesterol. Lifestyle also factors into cholesterol levels. Because so many factors come into play, your cholesterol management plan needs to be developed with your doctor's guidance. The American Heart Association endorses the National Cholesterol Education Program (NCEP) guidelines for detection of high cholesterol (see Appendix). Everyone age 20 and older should have a fasting "lipoprotein profile" every 5 years. This test is done after a 9- to 12-hour fast without food, liquids, or pills. It gives information about total cholesterol, LDL (bad) cholesterol, HDL (good) cholesterol, and triglycerides. If you are not fasting when the test is done, your doctor won't be able to get an accurate lipid profile and may need to test you again. Be sure to review your test results with your doctor so you can understand and follow your treatment plan.

You can't change your genetic makeup. Medication may be required to help manage your cholesterol. But remember, you always play a significant role in keeping your cholesterol under control.

84. What can I do about high blood pressure?

High blood pressure is often called the silent killer. Why? Because you can have high blood pressure and have no noticeable symptoms, but the accumulating damage can be life-threatening. When your blood pressure is too high, the heart has to work much harder to pump blood throughout the body. This can weaken the heart muscle. The pressure of your blood against the arteries can cause them to narrow and harden, putting you at risk for stroke, kidney disease, or heart attack. High blood pressure is anything over 140/90, although more and more doctors are beginning to express concern at numbers a little lower, with 120/80 or lower regarded as optimal.

As with other chronic conditions, some risk factors are not controllable and others are within your control. Race, family history, gender, and age are uncontrollable. But knowing your risk factors in these areas allows you to be proactive and take some preventive measures. Hypertension often develops earlier and with more ferocity in African Americans than in other races. African Americans are nearly twice as likely to suffer a fatal stroke, 1.5 times more likely to die from heart disease, and four times more likely to suffer kidney failure than are Caucasians. For black men, the picture is particularly disturbing—they face a death rate from disorders related to high blood pressure that's more than three times that of the death rate in white men.

There are factors that are within your control. Smoking raises blood pressure within 5 minutes and keeps it elevated for about 30 minutes, because nicotine causes the blood vessels to constrict. This same constriction happens with chewing tobacco. Smoking also interferes with some antihypertensive drugs, especially beta blockers. Excessive drinking—having three or more drinks per day—is a factor in about 7% of hypertension cases. It can also interfere with antihypertensive medications, increase your risk of stroke, and lead to heart failure. A wide variety of over-the-counter and prescription medications can cause elevated blood pressure. These include certain medications prescribed for autoimmune diseases, some cancer-treating agents, nasal decongestants, anabolic steroids, or MAO inhibitors (a class of antidepressants), as well as nonsteroidal anti-inflammatory drugs, or NSAIDs (Advil, Aleve). Decongestants found in many over-the-counter allergy, cold, and flu medications as well as weight-loss supplements can raise blood pressure and interfere with drugs used to treat it. You would be wise to discuss the use of any of these medications with your doctor if your blood pressure is even on the high side.

Remember that high blood pressure does not present symptoms until the damage is significant and irreversible. Not only does hypertension damage the blood vessels, it also damages the heart, brain, kidneys, and eyes. You want your blood pressure to stay under 120/80. Monitor your blood pressure regularly. Other lifestyle changes include cutting back on salt, losing excess weight, stopping smoking, limiting alcohol, eating a diet high in fruits and vegetables and whole grains, as well as regular exercise.

Remember that high blood pressure does not present symptoms until the damage is significant and irreversible.

85. What is obesity?

Sixty-six percent of adults in the United States are either overweight or obese. According to the Weight-Control Information Network, an informational service of the National Institute of Diabetes and Digestive and Kidney Diseases, obesity refers to an excessive amount of body fat, while overweight refers to an excessive amount of body weight that includes muscle, bone, fat, and water. Men with more than 25% body fat and women with more than 30% body fat are considered obese. The percentage of body fat is not the same as the body mass index. Some methods of measuring body fat are not practical for the average person. Two simple methods are often used: measuring the thickness of the layer of fat just under the skin in several parts of the body or sending a harmless amount of electricity through a person's body. The concentration of fat around the abdomen is a particular indicator of developing future obesity-related problems.

Obesity is the result of a number of factors. If you continually eat more calories than you burn, you will gain weight. Obesity tends to run in families, which means that obesity may come from genetics, diet and lifestyle, or a combination of both. Medications can cause significant weight gain. Thyroid disease can also cause obesity. Chronic illnesses may limit physical activity, resulting in added weight. Uncomfortable emotions like depression, anger, and feelings of isolation lead some people to eat to comfort themselves. More than likely, obesity is the result of a combination of these factors.

Environmental and social factors also contribute to obesity. Eating out, large meals, grabbing foods from vending machines that are high in fat and empty calories, along with lack of physical activity, result in people becoming obese. People living in poverty often choose high-calorie processed foods because they cost less than healthier foods. They may not have access to healthier choices either because of where they live or because of lack of transportation. In many poor neighborhoods you will have no problem finding a burger joint, fried chicken, or pizza place, but well-stocked grocery stores are nowhere to be seen.

86. Does obesity increase my risk of chronic disease or worsen existing chronic disease?

If you have a chronic disease and you are obese, you are likely to develop other chronic diseases. The chronic disease you already have will be much harder to manage. The following conditions or illnesses are the result of obesity.

- Coronary heart disease
- Type 2 diabetes
- Cancers (endometrial, breast, and colon)
- Hypertension (high blood pressure)
- Dyslipidemia (for example, high total cholesterol or high levels of triglycerides)
- Stroke
- Liver and gallbladder disease
- Sleep apnea and respiratory problems
- Osteoarthritis (a degeneration of cartilage and its underlying bone within a joint)
- Gynecological problems (abnormal menses, infertility)

87. What can I do if I am obese?

If your doctor has told you that you are obese, have a discussion with your doctor about the causes and solutions. The next and extremely important step is to decide that you can do something about your obesity. It's a difficult step. No one becomes obese because they want to be that way. You may feel like a failure, blame yourself, and feel hopeless and helpless. Develop a plan with your doctor or other specialist. Set small, clearly defined and reasonable goals. Saying that you are going to get more exercise is too vague, but deciding to walk 5 minutes a day is very clear. Set goals that you know you can achieve, rather than huge goals that seem unattainable at the moment. You want to build successes one at a time. Remember, you can always exceed your goal and feel good about it!

One tool to manage obesity is to make lifestyle changes. You may want to consult professionals to help you do this. Learn about good nutrition. The key to success is knowing just how calorie- and fat-laden some foods are and to make healthier choices. Create a diet and exercise plan. Try keeping a journal of what you eat and what physical activity you do each day. At the end of the day, review your journal. If you had difficulty following your plan, try to identify the obstacles, and think of ways to avoid or get around them if they occur again. Brainstorm with a friend, family member, or professional. Your lifestyle changes require changes in behavior. Regular meetings with a professional or support group will help you create success as the changes become part of your normal routine.

There are medications that may be able to help you lose weight. As with all medications, you will want to discuss risks versus benefits with your doctor. All medications have side effects. There is nothing magical about these medications. You will still need to make lifestyle changes. Bariatric surgery is an option for some people. More than 20% of people who have surgery for weight loss will have complications, but most complications are considered minor. Again, if you are considering this option, discuss it with your doctor. If you have other chronic illnesses, those need to be taken into consideration.

88. What is osteoarthritis?

Arthritis means inflammation or swelling of the joints and is usually painful to varying degrees. Rheumatoid arthritis is an autoimmune disease where the immune system mistakenly attacks and destroys the joints. Osteoarthritis is the result of aging, injury, or both. It is the most common form of arthritis. The ends of your bones are covered with cartilage, a hard but slippery surface that lets the bones glide over one another. The cartilage also acts like a shock absorber when you move. In osteoarthritis the cartilage breaks down and wears away. When the bones rub together the result is pain, swelling, and loss of motion. The joint may lose its normal shape. Bone spurs can form, break off, and float in the joint space, causing more pain and damage.

89. How can I manage osteoarthritis?

As with all chronic conditions, you play a major role in day-to-day management. People with osteoarthritis benefit from exercises that strengthen the muscles and support the joints. Weights or exercise bands increase resistance. Regular aerobic exercise is important for overall health. Range-of-motion and agility exercises help you continue to perform the activities of daily living. Always talk with your doctor before starting or changing your exercise program. Your doctor may recommend the use of over-the-counter pain medications or ice after exercising.

Maintaining a healthy weight will reduce the stress on your joints. Learn to pay attention to your body and stop or slow down when necessary. Regular periods of rest help prevent pain. Some people use canes, splints, or braces to take the strain off the affected joint. Keep in mind that you will still want to exercise the affected part; otherwise muscles will get lax, giving the joint less support.

Learn to pay attention to your body and stop or slow down.

Applying heat increases blood flow and eases pain and stiffness. Cold packs reduce inflammation and also lessen pain. Ask your doctor which approach is best for you. Massage also increases blood flow. Be sure to tell the massage therapist about any affected joints.

Your doctor may recommend over-the-counter pain medications or prescriptions. In some cases, surgery may be an option. The surgeon may remove loose pieces of bone and cartilage, reposition the bones, resurface or smooth out the bone, or replace the joint with an artificial one. Artificial joints can last 10 to 15 years or longer. The decision to use surgery takes into account age, occupation, level of disability, pain intensity, and the degree to which arthritis interferes with life for the patient. Rehabilitation follows surgery.

90. What is cancer?

Normal cells in everyone's body live for a certain pre-programmed period of time, die, and are replaced by new cells. When cells genetically mutate, this normal process can go wrong. Cells don't die when they are supposed to, and new cells are created when they are not needed. This can result in cancer. Cancerous cells can spread to nearby tissues and to all parts of the body.

According to the National Cancer Institute, an esti-mated 1,437,180 men and women (745,180 men and 692,000 women) will be diagnosed with, and 565,650 men and women will die of cancer in 2008. Not many decades ago cancer was considered a death sentence. Although people do still die from cancer, it is increas-ingly falling into the category of chronic illness as bet-ter tests for detection of cancer and better treatments are being developed.

91. How can I reduce my risk of developing a chronic disease?

There are three areas that need attention if you are to reduce your risk of developing a chronic disease or condition: know your risk, get tested, and be proactive.

Risk

Learn about personal risk factors that are beyond your control. Take the time to learn about the medical history of family members. Tendencies to develop some diseases are genetic. Be sure to inform your doctor about chronic diseases in your family tree. If you have a higher risk of cancer or hypertension or autoimmunity, you can be alert to changes in your health and take action quickly. Your ethnicity or race, gender, and age can predispose you to certain diseases. Although you can't eliminate this risk factor, you can eliminate risky behaviors associated with the diseases you are more likely to develop.

Get Tested

Follow the schedule of testing that your doctor recommends. When things like high blood pressure, diabetes, and cholesterol problems are detected in the earliest stages, treatment and management are most successful. If you are at risk for osteoporosis, have your bone density measured as your doctor suggests. It is far better to catch osteoporosis in the early stages than it is to end up with a hip replacement down the line. Have regular appropriate cancer screenings. Cancers caught early have a higher likelihood of cure than those that have progressed. Nancy Reagan said, "Don't fear the mammogram; fear the cancer." In other words, don't be an ostrich with your head in the sand. Just because you don't know you have a chronic illness brewing doesn't mean that it's not there!

Be Proactive

Care about yourself enough to take charge of your own health. No one else can do that for you. Here is a list of things that can help you reduce the risk of chronic illness.

Care about yourself enough to take charge of your own health.

- Know your risk factors
- Educate yourself about your health
- See your doctor regularly
- Get appropriate medical screenings
- Maintain a healthy weight

- Exercise to keep your heart healthy (cardio)
- Exercise to keep your muscles and bones strong (weight bearing)
- Exercise for flexibility (stretching)
- Don't smoke
- Limit alcohol intake
- Limit salt intake
- Eat whole, healthy foods
- Eat at least five servings a day of fruits and vegetables
- Avoid trans fats and dietary cholesterol
- Reduce stress where possible
- Manage stress that you can't avoid
- Practice living in the present
- Stay connected to other people
- Protect yourself from the sun
- Keep your immunizations up to date

PART ELEVEN

Looking Ahead

Where can I find a support network?

How can I find purpose and meaning in life again?

How can I stop myself from worrying about the future?

What is the difference between cure and healing?

More . . .

92. Where can I find a support network?

Support networks aren't found; they are created. You are the person who creates that network for yourself. When you have chronic illness, the tendency is to rely very heavily on those people closest to you—a partner, parent, child, sibling, best friend, or close neighbor. Remember that just as you are struggling with losses and changes in your life, your disease is causing losses and struggles in your friends' and families' lives, too. Does this mean you can't turn to them for support and help? Of course not! These people care about you, and they want to support you. But if you rely on one or two people to be your entire support network, sooner or later they are going to burn out. As many as 75% of marriages in which one partner develops a chronic illness or disability end in divorce.

Think about the types of support that you need. Be realistic about these things. Do you really need help? Is there some way you could modify an activity so that you could do it yourself? You may think you need help cooking, when what you really need is help chopping. Do you need help with activities of daily living? Shopping? Cooking? House cleaning? Driving? Do you need someone who you can talk to about your chronic illness experiences and frustrations? What else do you need? Now make a list of people who have offered to "be there for you." Next to each person's name write the way in which they can help you. Become aware of how often you have been turning to the same people. Spread your requests around. If you can't find people to support you, cast your net wider. Call a local church, synagogue, or mosque. Adults and teens are often available to help people who need it. Are there things that you could hire people to do? Maybe you can handle light housecleaning, but having a service come in once a month to do a more thorough cleaning would really help you.

For emotional support in coping with chronic illness you may have to look outside your usual resources. It can be very helpful to see a psychologist or social worker who has some experience with patients who have chronic conditions. Mental health professionals who work with oncology (cancer treatment) practices often have a very good understanding of the emotional and social problems that plague people with chronic conditions. It's not reasonable to expect your loved ones to fill this role. They are facing their own challenges in coping with your condition. Do talk to them, but also be willing to listen to how they are affected. You might both benefit by seeing the mental health professional together!

93. Where can I find a good support group?

The first step is to find a group, and the second is to figure out if it is a good group for you. You can find support groups by contacting the foundation that specializes in your particular disease. There is a foundation for almost every disease you can imagine. Many of them have support groups. Call your local hospital. Ask your doctor. Some psychologists offer groups. Check the health, club, or meeting information in your local newspaper's community calendar.

Before you can figure out whether or not a group is good for you, it is important to think about what you hope to gain from the group. Some people approach support groups thinking that they are like twelve-step groups. They think that they will be able to call other members of the group at any hour if they are feeling sad or frustrated. People in these groups are suffering with the same things as you. They are not likely to welcome a call at 3:00 a.m. because you are in pain, sad, or afraid. Others see support groups as a place to regurgitate their symptoms and problems. Doctors often hesitate to recommend groups because they perceive them as nothing more than suffering olympics and pity parties. This kind of group only makes people feel worse. Doctor-bashing is very common in these kinds of groups.

The best groups are those that do their best to remain positive. People are encouraged to share their experiences with the difficulties of illness, but not week after week after week! Once is enough. Good groups are places where other people with the same set of problems share solutions and coping strategies. Good groups are sources of reliable information. You will have to visit a group to truly get a sense of what goes on there. You might have to try more than one, but keep at it. If you walk out feeling worse than when you came in, the group is probably not for you. If you walk out feeling less alone, like there are other people who understand, and with information about how you can live more fully with your condition, then you have found a good group! And what if there are no groups or no positive groups where you live? Start one! There are other people just like you who wish there was such a group, and everyone is waiting for someone else to get it going.

94. How can I find purpose and meaning in life again?

People spend much of their lives searching for purpose and meaning. They craft their own personal direction gradually. Skills, work, productivity, and relationships all contribute to our identities. Then something uncontrollable—chronic illness—comes in and robs you of all the things that contribute to who you think you are. Nothing seems to matter. All is lost. Your old normal is gone. But you can build a new normal. You can create a new purpose and new meaning for your life. Finding purpose and meaning is a journey, not a destination.

Finding purpose and meaning is a journey, not a destination.

Realize that you are more resilient than you imagine. It's a good idea to take the time to write your thoughts and feelings as you read through the next few paragraphs. Writing makes the experience more concrete and helps to clarify your thinking. Think about all the difficult challenges you have ever faced and overcome. What did you do to live through ordeals and then get back to your life? What did you learn from these experiences?

Take a look at the tools you have for building a new life. How is your life with chronic illness different from your life before the illness? Make a list of all the things and abilities you have lost. Now make a list of all the things and abilities that you still have. You might want to do this over the course of several weeks. Sometimes it is helpful to ask a loved one to look over what you have written and make suggestions. When you are absorbed with your illness, it is hard to see the forest for the trees.

Accept the fact that change is part of living. Everyone changes. No one gets to stay the same. Some changes are beyond your control. Focus on the things that are within your control. Make realistic plans and short-term goals. Your goals should be something you want to do, not what other people think you should do. Be very specific defining a goal so that you will know with certainty when you have achieved it. If you don't have a lot of confidence that you will attain your goal, modify it so that you can do it. Be flexible, modifying your goals to reflect disease activity.

Stay connected with other people. You don't get to drop out of the human race because you have a chronic illness. Remember there are over 133,000,000 people just like you in the United States alone. Spend quality time with your loved ones. Be willing to ask for and accept help when you need it. Try new things. Most of all, remember that illness is a part of your life but not the center of it. You are not your illness.

95. How is journaling an effective tool in managing chronic illness?

Developing a chronic illness and then receiving a diagnosis along with the information that there is no cure, and that you will be stuck with this as long as you live, (or at least for a very, very long time) is traumatizing. Invasive medical tests and procedures are traumatizing. Stigma, loss of identity and self-esteem, and myriad unpleasant emotions are all companions of chronic illness. You may be inhibiting the expression of this trauma because you are afraid of acknowledging it or because you are afraid that you will alienate people who have to listen to you. In *Opening Up: The Healing Power of Confiding in Others,* James W. Pennebaker states that,

"Actively holding back or inhibiting our thoughts and feelings can be hard work. Over time, the work of inhibition gradually undermines the body's defenses. Like other stressors, inhibition can affect immune function, the action of the heart and vascular system, and even the biochemical workings of the brain and nervous systems. In short, excessive holding back of thoughts, feelings, and behaviors can place people at risk for both major and minor diseases."

You certainly don't need another disease, and you don't want to make the one you have worse. But you don't want to drive people crazy as you tell and retell your story. You may think that no one wants to be around a sick person. But as you just read, one way or another, the story and the feelings that accompany it have to be expressed. What can you do? You can journal. It's just as effective as telling your story to someone, maybe even more so.

Your journal can be written or you can speak it into a tape recorder. Either way, expressing what is on your mind can help you clarify your thinking and can have a profound influence on the way you see yourself and the impact of the disease on your life. When you talk or write about the trauma of chronic illness, you gain insights into yourself without the stress of inhibition.

96. How do I get started journaling?

The journal is your personal and private tool. It is not something you are going to share with others. You don't need to be concerned with grammar, spelling, punctuation, or penmanship. Your writing does not need to be structured like a formal essay. No one else is going to read and criticize what you write. What you want to do is get your thoughts on paper. The very process of doing that expresses feelings that you may have been inhibiting and gives you new insights into your relationship with your illness and life.

Get yourself a notebook if you plan to write your journal. My personal favorite is a half-size, college-ruled spiral notebook. You could get one of those pretty journal books, but remember, this is not about writing a romantic diary. It is about doing some hard work. What matters in journaling is that you just write down whatever comes to mind without regard to how the thoughts flow together. Just write. Write for at least 15 minutes. The only rule here is to keep the pen moving on the paper. Don't take time to sit and ponder unless you get a really big "ah-ha" insight. In that case, write it down before you forget your flash of insight. Pennebaker recommends that you write at least 4 days in a row for at least 15 minutes each time. You can write anywhere—at home, in a park, at a coffee shop, in an airport, whatever suits you. Different places stir up different thoughts.

Review your journal periodically. Rereading your journal entries 6 or more months after they were written is always revealing. Your journal becomes evidence of how far you have come. And knowing how far you have come, you find the strength to continue.

97. How can I stop myself from worrying about the future?

Most healthy people don't ever imagine that they might become sick or disabled.

Everyone's future is uncertain, no matter how much they prepare and plan. Most healthy people don't ever imagine that they might become sick or disabled. You probably didn't think it would happen to you. But it has happened to you. And it does happen to 3 out of 10 workers in the United States. Now that your illusion of a safe future has been shattered by chronic illness, your future looks much more frightening.

Dwelling in the future and imagining catastrophic scenarios only robs you of your present moments. Once those moments are gone, you can't get them back. Your future becomes a time of looking back, regretting the time you wasted worrying about the future. Of course, you know that you can't control the future. You can do things now that might influence it, but you can't control it.

When your mind runs off to the future or the past, there are ways to bring it back. If you have been meditating, you can recall the calm meditative state. If you haven't practiced meditation, you can still bring yourself back to the present. Stop for a moment, right now. Notice where your feet are and what they are touching. Become aware of the feeling of the air on your skin. Are you aware of your bottom seated in a chair? Are you warm or cold? Do you notice the texture of the paper and the cover of the book? What do you hear? Anytime you find your mind wandering off, you can bring it back by simply being aware of what is happening right at this moment.

If worries about the future persist, conduct a reality check. Ask yourself if anyone is threatening you right now. Are you undergoing a procedure right now? Are any of the things you are imagining happening right now? Do you have any real evidence that these things will happen? If you have a hard time doing this, check in with a friend or loved one. Ask them what they think. Then bring yourself back to the present.

If you are so agitated that you can't even apply these techniques, then count things. Name and count all the blue things in the room. Then do the same with red, green, orange, yellow, purple, black, and brown. Your mind can only really pay attention to one thing at a time. Once you begin to redirect your mind to the counting of different colored objects, you can go on to present-moment awareness and to challenging any irrational thinking.

98. What is an attitude of gratitude, and what difference will it make in my life?

"If you are breathing, then there is more right about you than there is wrong."—Jon Kabat-Zinn.

"If you are breathing, then there is more right about you than there is wrong."

Everyone, not just people with chronic illness, sometimes falls into the trap of taking the good things in life for granted. Instead they focus on the things that are wrong or not to their liking. The constant background noise of negativity creates stress, which makes you sick. You become more and more negative so that soon no one wants to be around you. You don't even want to be around yourself!

The goal here is not to become a Pollyanna who walks around saying, "Well, at least I don't have leprosy like that poor fellow." The goal is to become aware of what is actually happening in your life on a minute-by-minute basis. Try going through your morning routine and thinking about things in the way that follows. Of course, you will modify it to match your own life experience. Here are a few examples of ways to think about and be thankful for what you have in your life.

- Waking up: I am thankful that I sleep in a bed, that I have a roof over my head and walls around me, for the people who built this building, for the people who made the tools that were used, for windows and doors that keep out the elements, for pajamas, that I am breathing, that I know that I am awake, that I can feel parts of my body even if they hurt. What else comes to your mind?
- The bathroom: I am thankful that I have a toilet and don't have to go outside, for toilet paper, for people who make toilets and toilet paper, for the shower, for hot water, for people who work in well fields to bring me water, for those who maintain the pipes, for hot-water heaters, for electricity and gas, for the people who bring those to me, for soap and shampoo, for towels and wash cloths.
- What else comes to mind?

Try continuing this line of thinking throughout the day. Multitasking is a myth. Your mind focuses on one thing at a time. You will find, with practice, that you may even forget your illness for a few minutes. The stress of negativity will stop. Even if you don't believe all of this, just fake it till you make it. What do you have to lose?

99. What is mindfulness?

The majority of people spend most of their present moments with their minds in the past or the future. For people with chronic illness who are not as likely to be busy with the tasks of everyday living, it is even easier to have the mind anywhere but in the present. Mindfulness is a way of relating to what is happening in your life right in this present moment. When you practice mindfulness, you have a way of taking charge of your life and dealing with you illness. Over the past 28 years, the Center for Mindfulness at the University of Massachusetts has scientifically documented the benefits of mindfulness meditation. Their Web site states, "Restoring within yourself a balanced sense of health and well-being requires increased awareness of all aspects of self, including body and mind, heart and soul." Books have been written on mindfulness meditation from spiritual perspectives and from purely scientific perspectives. A lengthy discussion is outside the scope of this book. But if you'd like a little appetizer, visit the Center for Mindfulness online at www. umassmed.edu/Content.aspx?id=41252.

The majority of people spend most of their present moments with their minds in the past or the future.

You can try practicing mindfulness at home. Carve out some time for yourself, maybe 20 minutes. Turn off the phone, pager, TV, radio, and anything else that might distract you. Wear comfortable clothing. Sit or lie comfortably. Close your eyes. Simply notice your breathing. How does the air feel as it enters your body? Where does your body move as you breathe in? As you breathe out? Be still and follow the breath. Your mind will wander. Minds do that. Notice where the mind goes. Are you noticing discomfort or some other sensation in the body? Observe the fact that you were thinking and gently bring yourself back to the breath. Imagine a lake. Your thoughts are like bubbles that rise from the bottom of the lake. You can't hold onto them. Just observe the bubble or the thought passing. If you get restless or agitated, observe that too. But stay still, following the breath just a little longer. When you are ready, resume your normal activities.

You can also bring mindfulness to your daily activities. When you eat, eat slowly. Notice the temperature, taste, and texture of your food. When you comb your hair, pay attention to how your arm moves, to the feel of the comb on your scalp, to the movement of your hair. When you sit, notice the surface under you, what parts of your body are touching surfaces, pressure, the air touching your skin.

After some experimenting, you may decide to study mindfulness-based stress reduction in a more formal way. Many hospitals are now offering 8-week programs, and there are professionals around the country who can also instruct you. You can search for a local program through this link: www.umassmed.edu/cfm/mbsr/.

100. What is the difference between cure and healing?

We hope and pray for a cure. We explore alternative therapies. We surf the Web and hit the library. We latch onto any tidbit that we hear on the evening news that gives even the smallest ray of hope. We want our health back. We want to be cured. Most of us will never be cured.

Healing is different. Anyone can have it. You can have your disease and be healed at the same time. We are healed when we experience all the raw and painful emotions and let them go. We are healed when we learn to incorporate the disease into our lives without placing it at the center. We have a disease, and we can have a life too. For many people with chronic illness, the disease experience becomes a crucible, burning away all the useless things in their lives. Chronic illness can be a destructive fire or a refiner's fire. You get to choose. Healing empowers us to take responsibility for our health, to value each person and each minute, and to treasure everything we have.

Our wish for you is that this book will be a part of your journey to healing.

Doc Rob and Linda

Contact us at CopingWithChronicIllness@gmail.com

Follow Linda's blog at copingwithchronicillness.blogspot. com

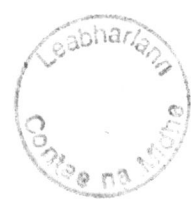

Aging with Dignity—Five Wishes
www.fivewishes.org
P.O. Box 1661
Tallahassee, FL 32302-1661
Phone: (850) 681-2010
Toll Free: 1-888-5WISHES (1-888-594-7437)
Fax: (850) 681-2481

Alcoholics Anonymous
www.aa.org
A.A. World Services, Inc.
P.O. Box 459
New York, NY 10163
Phone: (212) 870-3400

ALS Association (Lou Gehrig's Disease)
www.alsa.org
27001 Agoura Road
Suite 250
Calabasas Hills, CA 01301-5104
Phone: (818) 880-9007
Fax: (818) 725-9422

Alzheimer's Foundation of America
www.alzfdn.org
322 8th Avenue, 7th Floor
New York, NY 10001
Toll Free: 1-866-AFA-8484 (1-866-232-8484)
Fax: (646) 638-1546

American Association of Retired Persons
www.aarp.org
601 E Street NW
Washington, DC
Toll Free: 1-888-OUR-AARP (1-888-687-2277)

American Cancer Society
www.cancer.org
Toll Free: 1-800-227-2345

American Chronic Pain Association
www.theacpa.org
P.O. Box 850
Rocklin, CA 95677
Toll Free: 1-800-533-3231
Fax: (916) 632-3208

American Diabetes Association
www.diabetes.org
ATTN: National Call Center
1701 North Beauregard Street
Alexandria, VA 22311
Toll Free: 1-800-DIABETES (1-800-342-2383)

American Headache Society
www.achenet.org
19 Mantua Road
Mount Royal, NJ 08061
Phone: (856) 423-0043 Option 1
Fax: (856) 423-0082

American Heart Association
www.americanheart.org
American Heart Association National Center
7272 Greenville Avenue
Dallas, TX 75231
Toll Free: 1-800-AHA-USA-1 (1-800-242-8721)

American Liver Foundation
www.liverfoundation.org
75 Maiden Lane
Suite 603
New York, NY 10038
(212) 668-1000

American Lung Association
www.lungusa.org
1301 Pennsylvania Avenue NW
Suite 800
Washington, DC 20004
Toll Free: 1-800-548-8252

American Organ Transplant Association
www.aotaonline.org
21175 Tomball Parkway #194
Houston, TX 77070
Phone: (713) 344-2402
Fax: (713) 344-9422

American Psychological Association
www.apa.org
750 First Street NE
Washington, DC 20002-4242
Phone: (202) 336-5500
Toll Free: 1-800-374-2721
TTD/TTY: (202) 336-6123

American Self-Help Group Clearinghouse
www.mentalhelp.net/selfhelp/

American Spinal Cord Injury Association
www.asia-spinalinjury.org
2020 Peachtree Road, NW
Atlanta, GA 30309
Phone: (404) 355-9772
Fax: (404) 355-1826

American Stroke Association
www.strokeassociation.org
7272 Greenville Avenue
Dallas, TX 75231
Toll Free: 1-888-4-STROKE (1-888-478-7653)

American Thyroid Association
www.thyroid.org
6066 Leesburg Pike
Suite 550
Falls Church, VA 22041
Phone: (703) 998-8890
Fax: (703) 998-8893

Americans with Disabilities Act
www.ada.gov
Toll Free: 1-800-514-0301
TTY: 1-800-514-0383

Antiphospholipid Antibody Syndrome Foundation
www.apsfa.org
P.O. Box 801
LaCrosse, WI 54602-0801

Arthritis Foundation
www.arthitis.org
P.O. Box 7669
Atlanta, GA 30357-0669
Toll Free: 1-800-283-7800

Asthma and Allergy Foundation of America
www.aafa.org
1233 20th Street NW
Suite 402
Washington, DC 20036
Toll Free: 1-800-7-ASTHMA (1-800-727-8462)

Celiac Sprue Association
www.csaceliacs.org

Center for Mindfulness
www.umassmed.edu/Content.aspx?id=41252
University of Massachusetts Worcester Campus
Center for Mindfulness
55 Lake Avenue North
Worcester, MA 01655
Phone: (508) 856-2656

Centers for Disease Control—Obesity
www.cdcfoundation.org/healththreats/obesity.aspx
The CDC Foundation
55 Park Place, Suite 400
Atlanta, GA 30303
Phone: (404) 653-0790
Toll free: 1-888-880-4CDC
International: 00-11-1-404-653-0790
Fax: (404) 653-0330

Charcot-Marie-Tooth Association
www.charcot-marie-tooth.org
2700 Chestnut Street
Chester, PA 19013-4867
Phone: (610) 499-9264
Toll Free: 1-800-606-2682
Fax: (610) 499-9267

Chronic Fatigue and Immune Dysfunction Syndrome
www.cfids.org
CFIDS Association of America
P.O. Box 220398
Charlotte, NC 28222-0398
Phone: (704) 365-2343

Chronic Syndrome Support Association
www.cssa-inc.org
801 Riverside Drive
Lumberton, NC 28358-4625

Clinical Trials
www.clinicaltrials.gov

Co-Pay Assistance Programs
www.iononline.com/display.aspx?cid=CoPayAssistanceFoundations.cms

Crohn's and Colitis Foundation of America
www.ccfa.org
386 Park Avenue South
17th Floor
New York, NY 10016
Toll Free: 1-800-932-2423

Cystic Fibrosis Foundation
www.cff.org
6931 Arlington Road
Bethesda, MD 20814
Local: (301) 951-4422
Toll Free: 1-800-FIGHT CF (1-800-344-4823)

Endometriosis Foundation of America
www.endofound.org
872 5th Avenue
New York, NY 10065
Phone: (212) 988-4160

Epilepsy Foundation
www.epilepsyfoundation.org
8301 Professional Place
Landover, MD 20785
Toll Free: 1-800-332-1000

Exceptional Cancer Patients
www.ecap-online.org
ECaP 522 Jackson Park Drive
Meadville, PA 16335
Phone: (814) 337-8192
Fax: (814) 337-0688

Family Medical Leave Act
www.dol.gov/esa/whd/fmla/

HIPAA
www.hhs.gov/ocr/privacy/index.html

Hospice
www.hospicenet.org
401 Bowling Avenue
Suite 51
Nashville, TN 37205-5124
Check your phone book for your local Hospice office

International Oncology Network
www.iononline.com
3101 Gaylord Parkway
Frisco, TX 75034
Toll Free: 1-888-536-7696 Ext: 6847

Interstitial Cystitis Association
www.ichelp.org
100 Park Avenue South
Suite 108A
Rockville, MD 20850
Toll Free: 1-800-HELP-ICA (1-800-435-7422)
Fax: (301) 610-5308

Lupus Foundation of America
www.lupus.org
2000 L Street NW
Suite 710
Washington, DC 20036
Phone: (202) 349-1155
Toll Free: 1-800-558-0121
Fax: (202) 349-1156

Lyme Disease Foundation
www.lyme.org
P.O. Box 332
Tolland, CT 06084-0332
Phone: (860) 970-0070
Toll Free 24-Hour Hotline: 1-800-886-LYME (1-800-886-5963)
Fax: (860) 870-0080

Mayo Clinic
www.mayoclinic.com

Medicaid
www.cms.hhs.gov/MedicaidGenInfo
Toll Free: 1-877-267-2323
TTY Toll Free: 1-866-226-1819

Medicare
www.medicare.gov
Centers for Medicare & Medicaid Services
7500 Security Boulevard
Baltimore, MD 21244-1850
Toll Free: 1-800-MEDICARE (1-800-633-4227)

Medline Plus
medlineplus.gov

Multiple Sclerosis Society
www.nationalmssociety.org
Toll Free: 1-800-344-4867

Muscular Dystrophy Association
www.mda.org
Muscular Dystrophy Association–USA
National Headquarters
3300 E. Sunrise Drive
Tucson, AZ 85718
Toll Free: 1-800-572-1717

Myasthenia Gravis Foundation of America
www.myasthenia.org
355 Lexington Avenue
15th Floor
New York, NY 10017
Phone: (212) 297-2156
Toll Free: 1-800-541-5454
Fax: (212) 370-9047

Narcotics Anonymous
www.na.org
P.O. Box 9999
Van Nuys, CA 91409
Phone: (818) 773-9999
Fax: (818) 700-0700

National Alopecia Areata Foundation
www.naaf.org
14 Mitchell Boulevard
San Rafael, CA 94903
Phone: (415) 472-3780
Fax: (415) 472-5343

National Association of Area Agencies on Aging
www.n4a.org
1730 Rhode Island Avenue NW
Suite 1200
Washington, DC 20036
Phone: (202) 872-0888
Fax: (202) 872-0057

National Association of People with AIDS
www.napwa.org
8401 Colesville Road
Suite 505
Silver Spring, MD 20910
Phone: (240) 247-0880
Toll Free: 1-866-846-9366
Fax: (240) 247-0574

National Cancer Institute
www.cancer.gov
NCI Public Inquiries Office
6116 Executive Boulevard
Room 3036A
Bethesda, MD 20892-8322
Toll Free: 1-800-CANCER (1-800-422-6237)

National Center for Complementary and Alternative Medicine
nccam.nih.gov/
NCCAM Clearinghouse
P.O. Box 7923
Gaithersburg, MD 20898
Toll Free: 1-888-644-6226
International: (301) 519-3153
TTY: 1-866-464-3615
Fax: 1-866-464-3616

National Cholesterol Education Program
www.nhlbi.nih.gov/chd

National Chronic Fatigue Syndrome and Fibromyalgia Association
www.ncfsfa.org
P.O. Box 18426
Kansas City, MO 64133
Phone: (816) 737-1343

National Eye Institute
www.nei.nih.gov
2020 Vision Place
Bethesda, MD 20892-3655
Phone: (301) 496-5248

National Family Caregivers Association
www.nfcacares.org
10400 Connecticut Avenue
Suite 500
Kensington, MD 20895-3944
Phone: (301) 942-6430
Toll Free: 1-800-896-3650

National Graves Disease Foundation
www.ngdf.org
400 International Drive
Williamsville, NY 14221
Phone: (716) 631-2310
Toll Free: 1-877-643-3123
Fax: (716) 631-2822

National Heart, Lung, and Blood Institute
www.nhlbi.nih.gov
NHLBI Health Information Center
Attention: Web site
P.O. Box 30105
Bethesda, MD 20824-0105
If you are requesting health information, please include a current postal address,
   since many resources are available only as print publications.
Phone (301) 592-8573
TTY: (240) 629-3255
Fax: (240) 629-3246

National Institute of Arthritis and Musculoskeletel and Skin Diseases
www.niams.nih.gov
1 AMS Circle
Bethesda, MD 20892-3675
Phone: (301) 495-4484
Toll Free: 1-877-22-NIAMS (1-877-226-4267)
TTY: (301) 565-2966
Fax: (301) 718-6366

National Institute of Mental Health
www.nimh.nih.gov
Science Writing, Press and Dissemination Branch
6001 Executive Boulevard
Room 8184, MSC 9663
Bethesda, MD 20892-0663
Phone: (301) 443-4513
Toll Free: 1-866-615-6464
TTY Local: (301) 443-8431
TTY Toll Free: 1-866-415-8051
Fax: (301) 443-4279

National Institute of Neurological Disorders and Stroke
www.ninds.nih.gov
P.O. Box 5801
Bethesda, MD 20824
Phone: (301) 496-5751
Toll Free: 1-800-352-9424
TTY: (301) 468-5981

National Institute on Aging
www.nia.nih.gov
Building 31, Room 5C27
31 Center Drive, MSC 2292
Bethesda, MD 20892
Phone: (301) 496-1752
TTY: 1-800-222-4225
Fax: (301) 496-1072

National Institute on Alcohol Abuse and Alcoholism
www.niaaa.nih.gov
5635 Fishers Lane, MSC 9304
Bethesda, MD 20892-9304

National Institutes of Health
www.nih.gov

National Kidney Foundation
www.kidney.org
30 East 33rd Street
New York, NY 10016
Phone: (212) 889-2210
Toll Free: 1-800-622-9010

National Library of Medicine
Toll Free: 1-888-FIND-NLM (1-888-346-3656)
Local and International Calls: (301) 594-5983
Fax: (301) 402-1384
Interlibrary Loan Fax: (301) 496-2809
TDD access via Maryland Relay Service: 1-800-735-2258

National Mental Health Consumers Self-Help Clearinghouse
mhselfhelp.org
1211 Chestnut Street
Suite 1207
Philadelphia, PA 19107
Phone: (215) 751-1810
Toll Free: 1-800-553-4539

National Organization for Rare Disorders
www.rarediseases.org
55 Kenosia Avenue
P.O. Box 1968
Danbury, CT 06813-1968
Phone: (203) 744-0100
Toll Free: 1-800-999-6673 (voicemail only)
TDD: (203) 797-9590
Fax: (203) 798-2291

National Osteoporosis Foundation
www.nof.org
1232 22nd Street NW
Washington, DC 20037-1202
Phone: (202) 223-2226
Toll Free: 1-800-231-4222

National Parkinson Foundation
www.parkinson.org
1501 NW 9th Avenue/Bob Hope Road
Miami, FL 33136-1494
Phone: (305) 243-6666
Toll Free: 1-800-327-4545
Fax: (305) 243-6824

National Spinal Cord Injury Association
www.spinalcord.org
Toll Free: 1-800-962-9629

National Vitiligo Foundation
www.nvfi.org
P.O. Box 23226
Cincinnati, OH 45223
Phone: (513) 541-3903

National Women's Health Resource Center
www.healthywomen.org
157 Broad Street
Red Bank, NJ 07701
Toll Free: 1-877-986-9472
Fax: (732) 530-3347

NeedyMeds
www.needymeds.org
P.O. Box 219
Gloucester, MA 01931

NIH Senior Health
nihseniorhealth.gov

Partnership for Prescription Assistance
www.pparx.org
Toll Free: 1-888-4PPA-NOW (1-888-477-2669)

Patient Advocate Foundation
www.patientadvocate.org
700 Thimble Shoals Boulevard
Suite 200
Newport News, VA 23606
Toll Free: 1-800-532-5274
Fax: (757) 873-8999

Post Polio Health International
www.post-polio.org
(including Ventilator Users Network)
4207 Lindell Boulevard #110
Saint Louis, MO 63108-2930

Post Traumatic Stress Disorder Gateway
www.ptsdinfo.org

PubMed Central
www.pubmed.gov

Scleroderma Foundation
www.scleroderma.org
300 Rosewood Drive
Suite 105
Danvers, MA 01923
Phone: (978) 463-5843
Fax: (978) 463-5809

Sickle Cell Disease Association of America
www.sicklecelldisease.org
231 East Baltimore Street
Suite 800
Baltimore, MD 21202
Phone: (410) 528-1555
Toll Free: 1-800-421-8453
Fax: (410) 528-1495

Sjögren's Syndrome Foundation
www.sjogrens.org
6707 Democracy Boulevard
Suite 325
Bethesda, MD 20817
Toll Free: 1-800-475-6473
Local call: (301) 530-4420
Fax: (301) 530-4415

Smoking Cessation
www.smokefree.gov
Toll Free: 1-800-QUITNOW (1-800-784-8669)
TTY: 1-800-332-8615

Social Security Administration
www.ssa.gov
Toll Free: 1-800-772-1213
TTY: 1-800-325-0778

Stanford Chronic Disease Self Management
patienteducation.stanford.edu/programs/cdsmp.html
1000 Welch Road
Suite 204
Palo Alto, CA 94304
Phone: (650) 723-7935
Dedicated Spanish line: (650) 723-8165
Fax: (650) 725-9422

Tox Town
toxtown.nlm.nih.gov

Well Spouse Foundation
www.wellspouse.org
Toll Free: 1-800-838-0879

World Sleep Foundation
www.worldsleepfoundation.org

Appendix

Beattie M. *The Language of Letting Go.* New York: MJF Books/Hazelden; 1990.

Benson H, Klipper MZ. *The Relaxation Response.* New York: William Morrow & Company; 2000.

Benson H. *Beyond the Relaxation Response.* Zondervan: Grand Rapids, MI; 1984.

Berne K. *Chronic Fatigue Syndrome, Fibromyalgia, and Other Invisible Illnesses: The Comprehensive Guide.* Alameda, CA: Hunter House; 2001.

Borysenko J. *Guilt is the Teacher, Love is the Lesson.* New York: Warner Books; 1991.

Borysenko J. *Minding the Body, Mending the Mind.* New York: Addison-Wesley Pub./Bantam Books; 2007.

Baryshnikov J. *The Power of the Mind to Heal.* Carlsbad, CA: Hay House Inc.; 1995.

Boyd JH. *Being Sick Well: Joyful Living Despite Chronic Illness.* Grand Rapids, MI: Baker Book House; 2005.

Broyard A. *Intoxicated by My Illness.* New York: Ballantine Books; 1993.

Casey A. *Mind Your Heart: A Mind/Body Approach to Stress Management, Exercise and Nutrition for Heart Health.* New York: Free Press; 2004.

Cousins N. *Anatomy of an Illness as Perceived by the Patient: Reflections on Healing and Regeneration.* New York: Norton; 2001.

Donoghue P J, Siegel ME. *Sick and Tired of Feeing Sick and Tired: Living with Invisible Chronic Illness.* New York: Norton; 2000.

Dreher H. *The Immune Power Personality: Seven Traits You Can Develop to Stay Healthy.* New York: Dutton; 1996.

Fennell PA. *The Chronic Illness Workbook: Strategies and Solutions for Taking Back Your Life.* Delmar, NY: Spring Harbor Press; 2001.

Frankl VE. *The Will to Meaning: Foundations and Applications of Logo Therapy.* New York: Penguin; 1969.

Freeman A. *Woulda, Coulda, Shoulda: Overcoming Regrets, Mistakes, and Missed Opportunities.* New York: W. Morrow; 1990.

Goffman E. *Stigma: Notes on the Management of Spoiled Identity.* New York: Simon & Schuster, Inc.; 1963.

Graham-Pole J, Adams P. *Illness and the Art of Creative Self-Expression: Stories and Exercises from the Arts for Those with Chronic Illness.* Oakland, CA: New Harbinger Publications; 2000.

Greenberger D, Padesky C. Mind Over Mood: *Change How You Feel by Changing the Way You Think.* New York: Guilford Press; 1995.

Groopman J. *The Anatomy of Hope: How People Prevail in the Face of Illness.* New York: Random House; 2003.

Groopman J. *The Measure of Our Days: New Beginnings at Life's End.* New York: Viking; 1997.

Hanh TN. *Miracle of Mindfulness.* Boston, MA: Beacon Press; 1999.

Hanh TN. *Peace Is Every Step: The Path of Mindfulness in Everyday Life.* New York: Bantam Books; 1992.

Jacobs P. *500 Tips for Coping with Chronic Illness.* San Francisco, CA: Robert D. Reed Publishers; 1995.

John R, Williams P. *You Can't Afford the Luxury of a Negative Thought: A Book for People with Any Life-Threatening Illness—Including Life.* Los Angeles, CA: Prelude Press; 1988.

Kabat-Zinn J. *Coming to Our Senses: Healing Ourselves and the World Through Mindfulness.* New York: Hyperion; 2005.

Kabat-Zinn J. *Full Catastrophe Living: Using the Wisdom of Your Body and Mind to Face Stress, Pain, and Illness.* New York: Delacorte Press; 1990.

Kabat-Zinn J. *Wherever You Go, There You Are.* New York: Hyperion; 2005.

Kaschak E. *Minding the Body: Psychotherapy in Cases of Chronic and Life Threatening Illness.* New York: Haworth Press; 2001.

Kubler-Ross E. *On Death and Dying: What the Dying Have to Teach Doctors, Nurses, Clergy and Their Own Families.* New York: Scribner Classics; 1969.

Kushner HS. *Living a Life that Matters.* New York: Alfred A Knopf; 2002.

Kushner HS. *When Bad Things Happen to Good People.* New York: Schocken Books; 2004.

Lazarus J. *Stress Relief and Relaxation Techniques.* Lincolnwood, IL: Keats Publishing; 2000.

Lorig K, et al. *Living a Healthy Life with Chronic Conditions: Self-Management of Heart Disease, Fatigue, Arthritis, Worry, Diabetes, Frustration, Asthma, Pain, Emphysema, and Others.* Palo Alto, CA: Bull Publishing, Inc.; 2006.

Martin PR. *The Healing Mind: The Vital Links Between Brain and Behavior, Immunity and Disease.* New York: St. Martins Press; 1997.

Milstrey-Wells S. *A Delicate Balance: Living Successfully with Chronic Illness.* New York: Insight Books; 2000.

Moore T. *Care of the Soul: A Guide for Cultivating Depth and Sacredness in Everyday Life.* New York: Harper Collins Publishers; 1992.

Padus E, ed. *The Complete Guide to Your Emotions and Your Health: Hundreds of Proven Techniques to Harmonize Mind and Body for Happy, Healthy Living.* Emmaus, PA: Rodale Press; 1992.

Pennebaker JW. *Opening Up: The Healing Power of Expressing Emotions.* New York: Guilford Press; 1997.

Pennebaker JW. *Writing to Heal: A Guided Journal for Recovering from Trauma & Emotional Upheaval.* Oakland, CA: New Harbinger Press; 2004.

Pennebaker J, ed. *Emotion, Disclosure, and Health.* Washington, DC: American Psychological Association; 1995.

Pert C. *Molecules of Emotion: Why You Feel the Way You Feel.* New York: Scribner; 1997.

Pitzele SK. *We Are Not Alone: Learning to Live with Chronic Illness.* New York: Workman Publishers; 1985.

Pollin I, Golant S. *Taking Charge: How to Master the Eight Most Common Fears of Long Term Illness.* New York: Times Books; 1996.

Register C. *The Chronic Illness Experience: Embracing the Imperfect Life.* Center City, MI: Hazelden; 1999.

Rubin TI. *Overcoming Indecisiveness: The Eight Stages of Effective Decision Making.* New York: Harper & Row; 1986.

Selye H. *Stress Without Distress: How to Use Stress as a Positive Force to Achieve a Rewarding Lifestyle.* Philadelphia: Lippincott; 1974.

Siegel B. *365 Prescriptions for the Soul.* Novato, CA: New World Library; 2004.

Siegel B. *How to Live Between Office Visits: A Guide to Life, Love, and Health.* New York: Harper Collins; 1994.

Siegel B. *Love, Medicine, and Miracles.* New York: Harper & Row; 1988.

Spero D. *The Art of Getting Well: Maximizing Health and Well-Being When You Have a Chronic Illness.* Alameda, CA: Hunter House; 2002.

Svec C. *After Any Diagnosis: How to Take Action Against Your Illness Using the Best and Most Current Medical Information Available.* New York: Three Rivers Press; 2001.

Swedo SA. *It's Not All in Your Head: The Real Causes and Newest Solution to Women's Most Common Health Problems.* San Francisco, CA: Harper San Francisco; 1997.

Topf L. *You Are Not Your Illness: Seven Principles for Meeting the Challenge.* New York: Fireside; 1995.

Weill A. *Spontaneous Healing: How to Discover and Embrace Your Body's Natural Ability to Maintain and Heal Itself.* New York: Knopf; 2000.

Glossary

Aneurysm: Fluid-filled sac in the wall of a blood vessel that can weaken the wall and cause it to rupture.

Ankylosing spondylitis: An autoimmune disease that affects the spine and causes the bones to fuse together.

Artery: Blood vessel carrying blood away from the heart to the body.

Autoimmune disease: Any disease in which a person's immune system cannot tell the difference between viruses, bacteria, or parasites and the healthy self.

Biochemical: Relating to chemicals that are found in living organisms. Imbalances can cause disease and depression.

Cholesterol: A waxy substance found naturally in the body and necessary for some bodily functions. Cholesterol is also found in foods. An excess of cholesterol can cause buildup in the arteries, leading to hardening of the arteries and disease.

Chronic obstructive pulmonary disease (COPD): A disease of the lungs that hampers breathing and is often caused by smoking or exposure to inhaled chemicals.

Coronary artery disease: Disease of the blood vessels that involves the heart.

Crohn's disease: A chronic inflammatory disease affecting the digestive tract.

CT scan: A non-invasive medical test. CT imaging combines special X-ray equipment with sophisticated computers to produce multiple images of the inside of the body. These cross-sectional images of the area being studied can then be examined on a computer monitor or printed.

Diabetes (types 1 and 2): Diabetes occurs when the body is not able to keep blood sugar balanced. Type 1 diabetes is autoimmune. Type 2 diabetes develops as a result of obesity, lifestyle, or age.

End-organ toxicity: Problems that are caused by medication prescribed to treat another condition.

Epilepsy: A neurological condition that sometimes produces brief disturbances (seizures) in the normal electrical functions of the brain.

HDL: High-density lipoprotein, or "good" cholesterol.

HIV/AIDS: A virus-induced disorder of the immune system whereby a person loses the ability to fight infection.

Hypertension: High blood pressure.

Immunosuppressive drugs: Drugs designed to treat autoimmunity by weakening a person's immune system.

Isometrics: Exercises that involve pitting muscle against muscle or against an inanimate object (like a wall or door frame).

LDL: Low-density lipoprotein, or "bad" cholesterol.

Magnetic resonance imaging (MRI): A non-invasive medical test. MRI uses a powerful magnetic field, radio frequency pulses, and a computer to produce detailed pictures of organs, soft tissues, bone, and virtually all other internal body structures.

Multiple sclerosis: An autoimmune disease that affects the myelin sheath (covering) of the nerve pathways and disrupts communication to the muscles and other parts of the body.

Neurological disorders: Problems affecting the nervous system.

Neuropathy: Nerve pain.

Obesity: Overweight and obesity are both labels for ranges of weight that are greater than what is generally considered healthy for a given height. An adult who has a body mass index (BMI) between 25 and 29.9 is considered overweight. An adult who has a BMI of 30 or higher is considered obese.

Osteopenia: A slight or minor thinning of the bones.

Osteoporosis: Significant thinning of the bones requiring medical treatment.

Psoriasis: Chronic, autoimmune disease that appears on the skin. It occurs when the immune system sends out faulty signals that speed up the growth cycle of skin cells.

Psychiatrist: A mental health professional who can prescribe medication to treat mental and emotional problems.

Psychologist: A mental health professional who uses talk therapy and other techniques but does not prescribe medication.

Remitting/flaring: Periods of relative calm and periods of increased disease activity.

Rheumatoid arthritis: An autoimmune disease in which the immune system attacks and destroys the joints.

Index

economic status (*continued*)
    Partnership for Prescription Assistance
       and, 68
    Supplemental Security Income and, 67
elderly, chronic illnesses and, 4
electricity, body fat measurement and, 123
emotional support, 133
emotional suppression, chronic illnesses
    and, 78
empathy, social relationships and, 30–31
emphysema, 116
end-of-life issues, 45
endometriosis, 107
end-organ toxicity, medications and, 60
endorphins, 97
energy conservation, fatigue and, 73
environment
    obesity and, 124
    sleeping problems and, 87
epilepsy, 26
exercise(s), 15, 81–82
    cardiovascular, 82, 84
    depression and, 83
    diabetes and, 112
    isometrics and, 83
    Iyengar yoga, 83
    obesity and, 82
    for osteoarthritis, 127
        aerobic, 127
        agility, 127
        with bands, 127
        range of motion, 127
        weight-bearing, 127
    osteoporosis and, 114
    pain and, 77
    programs, 83–85
        goals and, 84–85
    resistance, 114
    sleeping problems and, 87
    strength, 83, 84
    stress and, 97
    stretching, 82–83, 84
    weight-bearing, 82, 83, 84, 114, 127
    yoga, 83
exercise bands, for osteoarthritis, 127

F

Family Medical Leave Act (FMLA), 39–41
    eligibility for, 40–41
fatigue
    goal achieving and, 73–74
    management of, 73–75
        energy conservation and, 73
        source identification in, 73

    from medications, 73
    pain and, 76
fault, grieving stages and, 12–14
fibromyalgia, 107
fight-or-flight response, 96
FMLA. *See* Family Medical Leave Act
Full Catastrophe Living: Using the Wisdom
    of our Body and Mind to Face
    Stress, Pain and Illness, 97

G

genetics
    cholesterol and, 121
    chronic illnesses and, 4
    obesity and, 124
gratitude, 139–141
Graves' disease, 109
grieving, stages of, 12–24
    acceptance, 19
    alienating others, 17
    anger, 16–17
        journaling and, 17–18
        management of, 17–18
    bargaining and, 23–24
    blame, 13–14
    denial, 15–16
    depression, 16
        biochemical, 21
        management of, 21–22
        psychiatrist for, 22
        psychologist for, 22
        symptoms of, 19–21
    fault, 12–14
    giving up, 18–19
    memory and, 22–23
    nutrition and, 15
    praying and, 23–24
    thought process and, 22–23
    why me, 12

H

Hashimoto's thyroiditis, 109
HDL. *See* high-density lipoprotein
healing, cure *vs.,* 142–143
health insurance
    disputes with, 57–58
    financial problems and, 66–68
    population without, 66–68
    Social Security Disability Insurance
       payments, 41–43
Health Insurance Portability and
    Accountability Act (HIPPA),
    43–44

Index